Dishes like these make it easy to move toward a low-fat lifestyle. And The Low-Fat Epicure *makes it even easier—with healthy eating guidelines, convenient nutritional information, and simple directions*
for . . .

PORTOBELLO MUSHROOMS TOPPED WITH
VEGETABLES AND FETA CHEESE
•
CHICKEN-YOGURT CURRY
•
CREAMY BROCCOLI SOUP
•
FRUITED CRANBERRY SALAD
•
MOIST CHOCOLATE CAKE
•
HEARTY BEEF STEW
•
LINGUINE WITH BROCCOLI AND
BLUE CHEESE SAUCE

and more . . .

The Low-Fat Epicure

THE

Low-Fat

EPICURE

Sallie Twentyman, R.D.

BERKLEY BOOKS, NEW YORK

THE LOW-FAT EPICURE

A Berkley Book / published by arrangement with
the author

PRINTING HISTORY
Berkley edition / June 1995

ISBN: 0-425-14687-1

BERKLEY ®
Berkley Books are published by The Berkley Publishing Group,
200 Madison Avenue, New York, New York 10016.
BERKLEY and the "B" design
are trademarks belonging to Berkley Publishing Corporation.

PRINTED IN THE UNITED STATES OF AMERICA

10 9 8 7 6 5 4 3 2 1

Contents

To my family: to my husband, Scott, without whose encouragement this book would never have been written; to my children, Elizabeth and Stephen, who have taught me to keep everything in perspective and never be too busy to spend time with those you love; to my mother and my two grandmothers, who taught me to love food; and to my father and grandfather, who always believed I could do whatever I set my mind to.

Acknowledgments

I wish to give thanks to the many people who encouraged me in writing this book and, more importantly, in pursuing my goal to prove that low-fat cooking *can* be delicious.

To my family and neighbors, especially Martha, Mike, and Emily Jolkovski, thanks for being such enthusiastic tasters, all the way from the first tries through the final testings. Your encouragement carried me through many days when I was tempted to do something a lot simpler for a living.

To my husband and friends, especially to my sister-in-law Dianne Spessard and Dr. Edward Curcio, thanks for helping me strive for what I want in life.

And a special thanks to my favorite food writers, whose books and articles I've dog-eared and studied throughout the years—especially Madhur Jaffrey's *An Invitation to Indian Cooking,* which taught me more about spices than I had ever known before; Barbara Kafka's "Opinionated Palate" columns in *Gourmet;* Elizabeth Rozin's *Ethnic Cuisine,* and, of course, *The Joy of Cooking,* whose pages taught me the basics of good cooking. Thanks, too, to Julia Child and to Rose Levy Beranbaum for their dedication to excellence. All of these people, through their writing, have taught me that recipes are very personal and written for real people, not simply for bookcases. They have inspired me to hang in there and do the very best that I can do.

Preface

Aside from my family, food was my first love in life. My mother was a wonderful cook who was known especially for her well-stocked pantry and freezer and for her ability to put together delicious home-cooked country meals on no more than a half hour's notice for anyone who dropped by. When I was a child, our home was always filled with wonderful aromas, as it seemed that she was always cooking.

Mom used only two recipes that I can remember, one for my grandmother's vanilla wafer cake and one for a family pound cake, both written out by hand on paper that was food-stained and crinkled with age. But she experimented daily, trying new combinations of whatever foods were available from the garden and farm and with whatever foods the budget allowed her to buy at the time. She turned most of those foods into delightful meals.

It was at home that I learned the real joy of cooking—foods that smelled delicious and greeted us with comfort when we walked through the door after a long day of work or play, foods raised and prepared with joy, foods to look forward to. Even in drought years on our farm, Mom filled our plates. My Dad, my brother, and I felt we had everything that was truly important in life, including wonderful food.

I never expected back then that I would be a good cook. It wasn't until years later, after I had left home and Mom's good food, that I realized I *had* to learn to cook. Childhood had taught me a love for food and for the warmth of the kitchen—a love that many of my friends didn't understand. I yearned to share it with them and recapture it for myself.

I began college as a physical education and mathematics major, but later changed to dietetics. I suppose now that I switched to the study of nutrition because it encompassed the worlds I loved best—food, science, people, and health. I now share my joy of food and eating with you in my own way, with an emphasis on eating for good health.

Introduction

I regard eating as one of the great pleasures of life. It is a pleasure I have no intention of giving up myself or of asking others to.

Dr. Richard Wolff, M.D., *Eating Right, Eating Well—The Italian Way*

I enjoy eating well, and I think that everyone should be able to enjoy good food. So when I became a registered dietitian, I felt a responsibility to do more than just help my patients understand the need to change the way they ate. I wanted to help them find ways to continue to enjoy their food.

My natural interest has always been in cardiac nutrition, since I grew up in a family with a lot of heart disease. But I also grew up with people who placed great value on enjoying good food, so I understood when my patients had a hard time adjusting to a life without butter, cream, red meat, and the fatty foods they had always loved so much.

One day I learned that *my* cholesterol was high, and that same year several of my relatives died from heart disease, one of them a cousin in his early forties. Then my own father was diagnosed with heart disease.

I realized that I had to change the way *I* ate. I hoped that, through changing my own lifestyle and cooking methods, I would learn firsthand how to help other people just like me and my loved ones to eat healthfully.

I did all of the things I advised my patients to do. I cut added fats like oil, butter, margarine, and shortening in half or more. I changed to low-fat milk and then to skim milk. I became an avid reader of food labels and bought low-fat substitutes for many of my high-fat favorites. I started sautéing in water and broth instead of fats.

But I also did more. I studied food science and worked out ways to eliminate fat altogether in a lot of my recipes. I also began insisting on fresh, top-quality ingredients whenever possible, because I learned that a lot less fat and salt were required to make these foods enjoyable.

My husband never noticed the reduction in fat, but he did notice that he enjoyed food more than ever. My friends agreed that my cooking tasted better than ever, and they wanted to know how I was doing it.

It was then that the idea for a newsletter was born. I planned the newsletter as a way to share my discoveries and recipes with others while also being able to stay at home with my two young children. After weeks of deliberating over a name for the newsletter, I finally settled on "The Low-Fat Epicure," hoping to share with others my philosophy that *it is possible to enjoy low-fat foods*. Since then I have tried to make the foods in the newsletter as enjoyable as possible because I feel that only by providing people with tasty recipes do we really help people to adjust to a low-fat lifestyle.

My patients, friends, and new subscribers were more than willing to give me advice. They wanted recipes that weren't difficult to prepare. They wanted some gourmet recipes, but, even more than that, they wanted recipes that they could enjoy every day—foods like chili, beef stew, brownies, and pizza. And they wanted foods that didn't sound or taste or look like diet food.

The recipes in this cookbook are lower in fat than those in most "low-fat" cookbooks. They are meant to help people who want to reduce the fat in their diet to no more than 20 percent of the calories from fat. Research has shown that this level is more effective in reducing atherosclerotic plaques, that it aids in long-term weight reduction, and that it reduces the risk of breast cancer. This level is also good for people who want lower-fat foods for everyday use so that they can occasionally enjoy their high-fat favorites without worrying about weight gain or their heart's health.

With this in mind, and with a strong commitment to making healthful food taste good, I now share these recipes with you. I hope they will help you enjoy healthful eating.

Nutritional Analyses

The nutritional analyses for recipes contained in *The Low-Fat Epicure Cookbook* were determined using Nutri-Calc HD software by CAMDE Corporation. This database uses the most current information from the USDA's Handbook #8 series, from Handbook #456, and from food manufacturers and producers.

Serving sizes were determined using guidelines set either by custom or by the Exchange Lists for Meal Planning. Adjust the size accordingly for smaller or larger appetites and for extra servings.

When a range is listed for an ingredient's amount, the first listed amount was used in the calculation. For example, if 2–3 Tbsp. is listed, 2 Tbsp. was used. If an ingredient is listed as optional, it was not figured into the calculation.

Exchange information is included for most recipes to help diabetics and people on weight-control diets. *Please realize that this does not automatically mean that all of the foods that include exchange information are suitable for diabetics, as some of the recipes do contain sugar and other simple sugars. Only you and your doctor can decide whether sugar is suitable for your individual diet.* Because everyone has individual medical and dietary needs, "The Low-Fat Epicure" and its staff do not intend to offer any medical advice. Always consult with your physician before changing your diet or beginning any weight loss or exercise program.

FAT CONTENT OF RECIPES

	Percentage Calories from Fat	
Food	Standard Recipe*	Low-Fat Epicure Recipe
Guacamole	72	0
Navy Bean Soup	31	5
Mushroom Soup	64	9
Spicy Chili	41	10
Chicken-Rice Soup	22	12
Potato-Scallion Soup	30	3
Macaroni and Cheese	46	15
Vegetable Lasagna	48	11
"Fried" Fish Squares	52	15
"French-Fried" Potatoes	47	16

| | Percentage Calories from Fat | |
Food	Standard Recipe*	Low-Fat Epicure Recipe
Old-Fashioned Coleslaw	66	3
Potato Salad	52	2
Blueberry Muffins	30	7
Banana Oatmeal Bread	38	6
Spoonbread	53	10
Drop Biscuits	42	20
Waffles	46	8
Carrot Cake	47	4
Peach Cobbler	21	1
Chocolate Cake	43	15
Hot Chocolate	45	7
Brownies	58	8
Creamy Cheesecake	63	27
Pumpkin Cake	45	7
Chocolate Chip Cookies	53	27
Oatmeal-Raisin Cookies	38	6
Lemon Meringue Pie	34	9
Berry Shortcake	39	3
Gingerbread	43	3

*Standard recipe values were estimated from nutritional value data obtained from the USDA Handbook #456; Bowes and Church's *Food Values of Portions Commonly Used*, 15th Edition; Krause's *Food, Nutrition, and Diet Therapy;* and Giant Food's *Eat for Health Food Guide*. Where values are not given for homemade products, values for commercial products were used.

· 1 ·

EATING FOR
GOOD HEALTH

Today, Americans are discovering that there's a lot more to "good eating" than simply eating lots of delicious foods—it's also eating foods that are good *for* us.

For some time now, we've known that the food that we eat can influence how healthy we are and how long we will live. Research shows that excess fat in our diet as well as excess weight increases our risk of heart disease. This has been a good incentive for a lot of people to learn a new style of eating.

Many other Americans, however, have given up their old eating patterns for reasons other than the fear of disease or death. They are making long-term changes because they FEEL so much better, have more energy, and enjoy life and their leisure activities more when they eat right.

Never has it been so easy to eat right. Nutritionists who used to focus on endless lists of "don'ts" now teach us that what's important is the proportions of foods that we consume. As long as we eat "in moderation" and "balance," there's no need to eliminate our favorite foods altogether. Chapter 4 will show that all it takes to change to a healthier style of eating is a little bit of knowledge and making some changes in the way you plan your meals, shop, and prepare your foods.

The Dietary Guidelines for Americans and the newer Food Guide Pyramid help us set goals and make food choices for a healthful eating style. They both focus on "moderation," the idea of enjoying all of our favorite foods, only consuming smaller quantities of the less healthful ones. It saves us from having to give up all of our favorite foods and keeps us from living in guilt whenever we do eat them. It lets us enjoy our food AND good health.

The recipes in this book follow these Dietary Guidelines, except that they are even lower in fat than the Guidelines' recommendations. That means that, if you use these recipes regularly, it is easy to add in your favorite foods and still meet the Guidelines for fat. If you have heart disease and your physician has told you to reduce your fat to 20% or less of your calories from fat, or if you wish to lower your fat intake to help with weight control, this book will help you live with your very low-fat diet without leaving you feeling deprived.

The Dietary Guidelines for Americans

1. EAT A VARIETY OF FOODS.

There are no perfect foods. Since most foods are high in some nutrients and low in others, it is best to mix foods. For instance, breads and grains are high in complex carbohydrates and B-vitamins, but are lacking in the vitamins A and C that are so plentiful in fruits and vegetables and in the calcium of dairy products.

Even within the same food groups, foods vary in nutritional content. For example, greens are high in vitamin A, whereas tomatoes are a good source of vitamin C. Therefore, it's best to eat a wide variety of foods.

2. MAINTAIN A HEALTHY WEIGHT.

The risk of developing several diseases, including heart disease, hypertension, hypercholesterolemia, adult-onset (or Type II) diabetes, and some types of cancer increase as people become overweight, and the risk grows higher as the weight gain continues. In many instances, blood cholesterol and blood sugar levels have returned to normal in people who have reduced their weight to healthful levels.

Charts can be helpful in finding your ideal (or "healthy") weight, but, since all bodies are so different, body fat measurements are better. More and more, health clubs and physicians are making body fat measurements available to their clients and patients. These tests are the only way to know for sure whether you are "overfat"; some athletes are "overweight" but, because muscle weighs more than fat, they actually have more muscle and a lot less fat than their lighter friends.

Research has shown that where your extra fat is located can itself be an indicator of whether your extra pounds put you at increased risk for developing obesity-related diseases. The "pear-shaped" person (who carries extra weight primarily in the hip area) seems to be at a lower risk for disease than someone with an "apple-shaped" figure (with their extra weight at their waist).

A simple way to test whether your weight poses a special risk for disease for you is to measure your waist (area with the smallest circumference near your navel) and your hips (area of largest circumference between your waist and knees). Divide the waist by the hip measurement. If the circumference is greater than 1.0 for men or 0.8 for women, then you may be at increased risk for developing obesity-related diseases such as heart disease and diabetes.

3. CHOOSE A DIET LOW IN FAT, SATURATED FAT, AND CHOLESTEROL.

The American Heart Association and the National Research Council now recommend a diet in which fat provides 30 percent or less of its calories from fat with 10 percent or less of the calories coming from saturated fat. Cholesterol should be limited to 300 mg a day. Some experts are advising people with active heart disease to decrease fat intake to 20 percent or less of calories from fat.

Increased serum cholesterol is a risk factor for heart disease. The present "safe limit" is set at 200 mg/dl,* and anyone with a higher value is considered at increased risk for heart disease. Some cardiologists suspect that this safe limit of 200 should be lowered to 180 or even lower, since the rate of heart disease

*These are the standard units that laboratories use in measuring the amount of cholesterol in the blood.

tends to be much lower in individuals with lower cholesterol values.

The best dietary regimen for lowering blood cholesterol is a low-fat diet, especially one low in saturated fat. For more information on dietary recommendations for heart disease, see chapter 2.

Research is also showing that high-fat diets are a risk factor for developing some types of cancer, especially breast cancer. And certainly low-fat diets help with long-term weight control (see chapter 3). As mentioned before, weight control itself is very important for maintaining good health.

4. CHOOSE A DIET WITH PLENTY OF VEGETABLES, FRUITS, AND GRAIN PRODUCTS.

Vegetables and fruits are rich in vitamins, minerals, and fiber. They are the main dietary source of vitamins A and C along with some B-vitamins, and they also provide some iron and calcium. They are virtually fat free and supply fewer calories than any other food group. Grain products are also rich in B-vitamins, fiber, and complex carbohydrates.

5. USE SUGARS ONLY IN MODERATION.

Research today suggests that sugar itself is not harmful to the body except in the presence of blood glucose metabolism disorders such as diabetes. However, sugar contributes only empty calories to the diet, meaning it supplies calories without any protein, vitamins, minerals, or fiber. Because of this, it can contribute to unnecessary weight gain, especially in adults. In addition, sugar contributes to the development of dental caries, and some people report mood swings or conditions commonly referred to as "sugar addictions" when they consume foods high in sugar. Therefore, it is best to focus on eating the foods that contribute to our good health and to keep our use of sugar to a minimum.

6. USE SALT AND SODIUM ONLY IN MODERATION.

Sodium has been shown to increase blood pressure and to cause fluid retention in some people, making it wise for most people to use salt only in moderate amounts. Since table salt (sodium chloride) is the major source of sodium in the American diet, people should reduce the amount of salt used in food preparation and limit the amount of salty foods they eat.

7. IF YOU DRINK ALCOHOLIC BEVERAGES, DO SO IN MODERATION.

Despite the recent research suggesting that limited amounts of red wine may help to decrease the risk and incidence of heart disease, it is still wise to avoid heavy use of alcoholic beverages so as to reduce the risk of other health problems such as liver and pancreatic disease and some glucose intolerances, especially for those who use insulin. Also, alcohol, like sugar, supplies only empty calories. Each gram of alcohol supplies 7 calories in comparison to only 4 calories per gram of carbohydrate and protein and 9 calories per gram for fat.

Keep in mind, however, that alcohol can be used in cooking to flavor foods so that you do not need as much salt and fat. Much of the alcohol itself evaporates during cooking—especially when the food is cooked uncovered for a long time—leaving only the flavor behind.

The Food Guide Pyramid

In 1992 the U.S. Department of Agriculture designed a new food guide pyramid to help take the confusion out of eating right. Before that time, we were taught to eat some foods from each of the basic four food groups every day. The new pyramid, on the other hand, gives us a visual model of an eating style that meets the dietary guidelines without our having to remember rules or a long list of do's and don'ts.

In the food guide pyramid, foods are divided into five major groups. The foods that should form the foundation of our diet are placed at the bottom of the pyramid. Other foods that should also be included in smaller amounts are placed farther up the diagram.

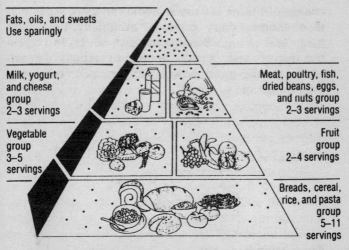

Fats, oils, and sweets
Use sparingly

Milk, yogurt, and cheese group
2–3 servings

Meat, poultry, fish, dried beans, eggs, and nuts group
2–3 servings

Vegetable group
3–5 servings

Fruit group
2–4 servings

Breads, cereal, rice, and pasta group
5–11 servings

Figure 1. The Food Guide Pyramid

To ensure an intake that is low in fat—especially in saturated fat—and high in fiber, build your meals and snacks around grains and breads and fruits and vegetables, all of which are near the bottom of the pyramid, and serve smaller amounts of meats and dairy products. Use sweets and fats sparingly.

This style of eating limits not only fats but also calories, making it easier to maintain a healthy weight. To plan your own weight control program without dieting, strive to eat the foods recommended by the pyramid in the suggested number of servings. Limit fats and sweets to a minimum (see chapter 3).

Check to see how your diet stacks up to the recommendations. Take a day, and check off the boxes in Figure 2 (one box per serving) for all the foods that you consume. Then you can see where you meet—or fall short of—the goals.

If you need to make some changes, go slowly and change one thing at a time—adding an extra vegetable, then another dairy product, eventually using less meat, and so on. Changing too fast can lead to digestive distress and, in many people, to feelings of deprivation. Going more slowly can give your body *and* your mind time to adjust.

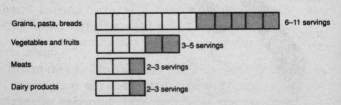

Figure 2. Record Chart

To receive a free copy of the thirty-page pamphlet "The Food Guide Pyramid," write to the U.S. Department of Agriculture, 6505 Belcrest Road, Hyattsville, MD 20782.

Daily Serving Guide

BREADS, CEREALS, RICE, AND PASTA: 6–11 servings. One serving: 1 slice bread; 1 oz. ready-to-eat cereal; or ½ c. cooked cereal, rice, pasta, or other grain

VEGETABLES: 3–5 servings. One serving: 1 c. raw leafy vegetables; ½ c. other vegetables, cooked or raw; ¾ c. vegetable juice

FRUITS: 2–4 servings. One serving: 1 medium piece fresh fruit: ½ c. raw, cooked, or canned fruit; ¾ c. fruit juice

DAIRY PRODUCTS: 2–3 servings. One serving: 1 c. milk or yogurt; 1½ oz. natural cheese; 2 oz. processed cheese

MEAT, POULTRY, FISH, DRIED BEANS, EGGS, AND NUTS: 2–3 servings. One serving: 2–3 oz. cooked lean meat, poultry, or fish. *Note:* ½ c. cooked dried beans, 1 egg, or 2 tbsp. peanut butter count as 1 oz. of lean meat

FATS, OILS: Use sparingly. One serving: 1 tsp. margarine, butter, or oil; 2 tsp. diet tub margarine; 1 tbsp. regular salad dressings; 1 serving of snack food containing 5 grams fat

SWEETS: Use sparingly. One serving: 1 slice angel food cake, ½ c. frozen yogurt or low-fat frozen dairy dessert, 2 medium-sized cookies, 1 small slice unfrosted cake, or 1 serving any dessert from "The Low-Fat Epicure"

· 2 ·

EATING FOR A
HEALTHY HEART

Each year more than a million Americans suffer heart attacks and half a million die of coronary heart disease. Each of us can take action to reduce our risk of being included in these alarming statistics. We can start by watching the foods we eat—especially the kinds and amount of fat in our foods. But before we try to understand how diet can affect our heart's health, it's a good idea to understand a little about the nature of heart disease.

Most coronary heart disease (CHD) is caused by atherosclerosis, a progressive disease that develops when cholesterol (a waxy white substance present in the cell membranes of animals) and fats build up on the inside of arterial walls. When these deposits become large enough, they cause bulging and hardening inside the arteries, and blood cannot flow as efficiently. This impaired blood flow causes the weakness and shortness of breath often seen in heart disease.

When the narrowing becomes extensive enough, the blood supply can be cut off completely, usually by a blood clot or coronary-artery spasm, causing a myocardial infarction, or heart attack. Such a blockage in the brain results in a cerebral infarction, or stroke. Regular checkups can sometimes diagnose heart disease at an early stage when it is easier to treat.

Many risk factors such as cigarette smoking, high blood pressure, and a family history of heart disease contribute to the development of heart disease. We cannot change some risk factors such as age, sex, and genetic makeup, but high blood cholesterol is one major risk factor over which we do have some control.

Most people can reduce their blood cholesterol by making some changes in the way they eat and by increasing their activity levels. This is important, because it is estimated that for every 1 percent decrease in blood cholesterol levels, there is a corresponding 2 percent decrease in risk of heart attack. Low-fat, low-cholesterol diets can decrease serum cholesterol levels by up to 15 percent or more. In studies conducted by Dr. Dean Ornish of the University of California at San Francisco, some people reversed their atherosclerotic plaques and heart disease by following a vegetarian diet with only 10 percent of their calories coming from fat and with a negligible cholesterol intake. Obesity can raise blood cholesterol, and even small amounts of weight loss in people who are overweight can reduce cholesterol levels. Exercise is also important and can make dietary changes even more effective.

The National Institutes of Health estimate that more than 50 percent of adults twenty years old or older have blood cholesterol values equal to or greater than 200. Desirable levels have been set at less than

200 mg/dl, with levels of 240 mg/dl being considered very high. Other cardiologists feel that the safe level should be lowered to 180 mg/dl or lower since the rate of heart disease is significantly reduced in persons with this lower cholesterol level.

We now know that we need to do more than simply check our total cholesterol level, as there are two major kinds of cholesterol in our blood—one that's not so good for us and another that is actually protective. LDLs (low-density lipoproteins), often referred to as the "bad cholesterol," are the form in which most cholesterol is carried in the blood. HDLs (high-density lipoproteins), the "good cholesterol," seem to transport cholesterol from the blood back to the liver, where it can be removed from the body.

A lipid profile is the best way to check to see whether your cholesterol level is a risk for you. If your profile shows a higher than normal LDL level (above 130 mg/dl) or a low HDL level (below 35 mg/dl), you need to take steps to reduce your cholesterol risk.

So how should we eat to lower our cholesterol? Lowering our saturated fat consumption seems to be the most important step we can take to prevent the buildup of atherosclerotic plaques. Lowering our cholesterol and overall fat intake is important as well. To prevent atherosclerotic disease, the National Cholesterol Education Program suggests that all Americans eat a diet in which less than 10 percent of a day's calories come from saturated fat and less than 30 percent from total fat; 300 mg dietary cholesterol a day should be the limit.

What does this mean? It means eating less total fat, especially fat from animal and dairy sources (saturated fats). Fats that are solid at room temperature—meat drippings, butter, and hydrogenated vegetable fats, for example—are usually more saturated than those fats that are liquid, such as oils. When fat is needed, it is best to use polyunsaturated fats such as safflower, corn, soy, cottonseed, sesame, and sunflower oil, or monounsaturated fats such as olive or canola oil. Some recent research suggests that monounsaturated fats may reduce LDL levels without influencing the HDLs, so it may be wise to include monounsaturated fats in the diet.

Reducing your cholesterol intake by limiting yourself to 3 or 4 egg yolks a week and by eating fewer organ meats and other high-cholesterol foods is also a good idea. Remember that foods high in saturated fat are often also high in cholesterol. Research shows a relationship between soluble fiber intake (oat, rice, and soy bran as well as dried beans and apple fiber) and decreased cholesterol levels, so be sure to include lots of whole grains and beans in your diet. Since weight control is important in controlling blood lipids, avoid foods high in simple sugars (sweets), which contribute calories without other desirable nutrients.

Other studies suggest that it is not simply blood cholesterol but the oxidation of this arterial cholesterol by free radicals that leads to heart disease. If this is so, then vitamin C, vitamin E, and beta-carotene (vitamin A), of which fruits and vegetables are excellent sources, may help prevent this oxidation. This is another good reason to aim for the five or more half-cup servings of fruits and vegetables a day that the National Academy of Sciences currently recommends.

So how does the typical American diet stack up to

these recommendations? Not well, it seems. Estimates indicate that 37 percent to 40 percent of our calories come from fat. This book will give you alternatives to high-fat foods. It also includes low-fat recipes for many of your favorite foods.

As you study your diet, remember that it is impossible to evaluate your overall daily fat intake by singling out particular foods. To check your own diet, record all the foods you consume in a day along with the fat content for each of the foods. You'll find the fat content of each individual food on the label or on one of the fat-counter guides available at bookstores. At the end of the day, add the fat grams together to get a total, and compare your score to the table below:

DAILY CALORIE AND FAT INTAKE

Recommended daily caloric intake	Daily fat allowance (in grams) if 30% calories from fat	Daily fat allowance (in grams) if 20% calories from fat
1,200	40	27
1,500	50	33
1,800	60	40
2,100	70	47
2,500	83	56

Most groups recommend using the 30 percent rule, but some current research is suggesting that an even lower amount of fat may help people who have heart disease. If you currently have heart disease, or if you want to lose weight, you may want to limit your fat intake to 20 percent of calories.

If your recommended caloric intake is not listed in the table above, use this formula:

For 30% rule: Maximum fat intake in grams = recommended caloric intake for day ÷ 30

For 20% rule: Maximum fat intake in grams = recommended caloric intake for day ÷ 45

The National Institutes of Health distribute an excellent publication entitled "Facts about Blood Cholesterol." You can receive a free copy by writing to the National Cholesterol Education Program Information Center, 4733 Bethesda Avenue, Suite 530, Bethesda, MD 20814-4820.

· 3 ·

EATING FOR LONG-TERM
WEIGHT CONTROL

Many people dream of losing weight and keeping it off. In fact, Americans have spent billions of dollars on diet programs that promise to help them lose a lot of weight quickly and permanently. But most of these programs haven't worked. In fact, studies show that Americans today are heavier than ever and that, if anything, all of their dieting during the past twenty or thirty years has only made matters worse.

Indeed, research shows that yo-yo dieting—frequently losing and regaining weight—can be risky business and that the more we diet, the harder it is for us to lose weight. Each time we diet, our metabolism slows down a bit so that instead of losing weight we burn fewer calories. Hormone levels can change, causing us to deposit fat more easily than before we started to diet. Some scientists now feel that it is healthier to weigh a little more and diet less.

However, extra pounds do pose a health risk, including a higher risk of heart disease, adult-onset (or Type II) diabetes, gallbladder disease, and orthopedic problems, to name a few. So what can we do to lose weight healthfully?

23

First of all, decide whether you really need to lose weight. Many American women *want* to weigh about 10 pounds less than their ideal weight. The exaggerated thinness that is exalted by the media is not a reasonable goal for most people—certainly not for those in their thirties and forties.

Weight charts can be deceptive, too, because people all have different body types. An example is a naturally muscular person who has a very low body fat; it's possible for him to weigh more than someone else with small muscles and more fat. The best way to know for sure whether you really need to lose weight is to have a body composition or "body fat analysis" done. That will tell you whether you're truly overfat. Ask your physician, registered dietitian, or health club director where you can have a body composition analysis done in your area.

To see whether your fat distribution puts you at increased risk for developing obesity-related diseases, you can do the measurement test described under "Dietary Guidelines" in Chapter 1.

If you determine that you really do need to lose weight, commit yourself to making long-term lifestyle changes. Weight gain doesn't happen overnight, and it's not healthy to lose it that quickly, either. Most nutritional authorities now recommend that you start counting fat grams instead of calories. This can bring about gradual weight loss while also promoting good health—and extra flexibility.

How does this work? When you consider that 1 gram of fat adds a whopping 9 calories to the diet, as opposed to 4 calories from protein and carbohydrate, it's easy to see why decreasing the amount of fat also automatically cuts the calories and makes it easier to lose weight. At the same time, there are plenty of low-fat foods left to supply us with the energy we need and to keep our metabolism working at regular speed.

Some studies suggest that low-fat diets work for reasons other than simply lowering the calories. Fat seems to be more easily deposited as body fat than are carbohydrates or protein—in other words, people gain weight faster on high-fat diets than on low-fat, high-carbohydrate diets with the same number of calories. The body deposits fat most efficiently in the presence of lipoprotein lipase, an enzyme released in larger amounts when we eat fat.

Many people, especially men, can lose weight simply by cutting the fat, not the volume of food. It's possible to lower the fat in your foods quickly by making just a few changes in the way you prepare and eat them. Bake or broil meats without fat instead of frying or sautéing them. Leave off fat-laden sauces, or make them lower in fat. Omit or reduce the amount of butter or margarine on vegetables and breads. Use lower-fat or fat-free dairy products. Remember that each teaspoon of oil, margarine, or butter supplies 5 grams of fat, or 45 calories. While one type of oil may be better for you than another—polyunsaturated or monounsaturated is preferable to saturated, for example—they all contain the same amount of fat and calories. Some margarines have had water or other fat-free ingredients added to them to dilute the fat, so be sure to read the labels for their fat content. (See chapter 4 for information about how to make these changes.)

If lowering the fat a little isn't enough to help you lose weight, try lowering it further, to 15 or 20 percent calories from fat, and get more exercise. Also watch your sugar intake and portion sizes of breads and starchy foods like potatoes, pasta, rice, and corn. For advice on how to restructure your eating pattern to lose weight without dieting, see the section below.

Changing Your Eating Pattern to Lose Weight

The USDA's Food Guide Pyramid (see Figure 1) was developed to help guide us toward better eating habits. When used properly, it can also serve as a basis for a safe and effective long-term weight-loss program.

The food pyramid breaks foods down into six groups and specifies the recommended number of servings for each group.

It makes sense to follow this model for healthful eating when you're trying to lose weight. By focusing on eating the recommended foods and eliminating extra foods and extra servings, you can lose weight safely and healthfully. To see how this can work for you, follow the guidelines below.

Note: Check with your physician before beginning any weight control program.

1. Set a suitable calorie level for weight loss. Weight loss should occur at a rate of no more than 1–2 pounds a week after the first two weeks. Losing weight faster than this can lead to dehydration, electrolyte imbalance, and muscle loss.

An easy method for setting a calorie level is to take your ideal body weight and add a zero—for example, if your ideal weight is approximately 140 pounds, then try 1400 calories as a daily calorie level.

Most registered dietitians and nutritionists do not

suggest going much below 1400–1500 calories per day, as it is very difficult to meet your daily nutritional needs on fewer calories than this. Also, a lower calorie level than this is likely to slow down your metabolism and increase your levels of lipoprotein lipase, an enzyme that promotes fat storage, making weight loss even more difficult later on. If you cannot lose weight on 1400–1500 calories, step up your exercise level before dropping the calories any further.

2. Use the Daily Servings table in Figure 3, below, to choose the number of servings from each food group that will provide the number of calories you have chosen. Transfer the appropriate numbers to a copy of the Record Chart in Figure 2.

DAILY SERVINGS

	Grains, pasta, breads	Vegetables, fruits	Meats	Dairy products	Fats	Sweets
1300 cal	6	5	5	2	1	0
1400 cal	6	5	5	2	2	½
1500 cal	6	6	5	2	2	1
1600 cal	6	7	5	2	3	1
1700 cal	7	7	5	2	3	1
1800 cal	8	8	5	2	3	1
2000 cal	9	8	5	3	4	1

Figure 3. Daily Servings for Weight Control

3. Shade in or cross out any extra boxes on your Diet Checklist to leave you with a personal chart for your daily record. Make extra copies so that you can have a new chart each day.

4. As you eat your meals each day, check off a

block next to the food group that matches up with each food you eat—¾ c. orange juice, for example, equals one fruit. When you reach the end of your boxes, that is your maximum for that food group for the day. If you are still hungry, it is best to eat more fruits and vegetables rather than foods from the other groups. Foods from this food group are lower in calories than those from the other groups, and these foods are practically fat free.

Learn to rearrange your food choices to meet your daily goals. For instance, if you plan to go out for a large dinner, eat a lighter lunch so that you'll have more servings left for your dinner.

5. If you add fat to any of your foods, be sure to record it under the fat group. Remember that 1 fat equals 5 grams of fat. If you eat a prepared food such as potato chips, read the label to see its fat content. Since potato chips contain 10 grams of fat per ounce, count one 1-oz. serving as 2 fats for the day.

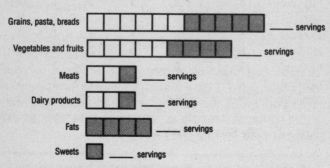

Figure 4. Diet Checklist

6. If you consistently eat too much of one group or too little of another, think of ways to include more of the recommended foods and fewer of the others. If you continue to have problems, schedule an appointment with a registered dietitian to help set up a plan that is right for you.

7. Remember that exercise is an important part of any weight-loss program. Statistics show that people who exercise when losing weight are much more successful at keeping the weight off. Not only do they burn extra calories, but they also help ensure that their weight loss comes mostly from fat. Without this exercise, the dieter loses some muscle mass, too. Since the number of calories your body needs for fuel depends on the amount of muscle you have, your metabolism increases when you exercise.

Exercise also promotes a sense of caring for your body and reduces stress and stress-induced eating. But *always check with your physician before beginning any new exercise program*.

The lowest calorie level is 1300. It is impossible to meet the Food Pyramid Guide recommendations in fewer calories than this.

I have grouped fruits and vegetables together to allow for more flexibility; however, remember that it is important that you regularly include both in your daily diet. Also, I have added a "Sweets" category to help you avoid the feelings of deprivation that can sabotage your weight-loss efforts. Just be sure to eat sweets in the serving sizes listed.

Sample Menu
Example: 1500 calories

BREAKFAST
1 whole English muffin (2 grains)
2 tsp. diet tub margarine (1 fat)

½ c. orange juice (1 fruit or vegetable)
Black coffee (free)
1 c. skim milk (1 dairy)

SNACK

1 small apple (1 fruit or vegetable)
Diet coke (free)

LUNCH

Turkey sandwich made with 2 oz. turkey, 2 slices bread, tomato, lettuce, onion (2 oz. meat, 2 grains, 1 fruit or vegetable)
Lettuce salad with fat-free dressing (1 fruit or vegetable)
Mixed fruit salad (1 fruit or vegetable)
Iced tea with lemon (free)

SNACK

8 oz. fat-free yogurt (1 dairy)

DINNER

3 oz. chicken skinless baked breast (3 oz. meat)
½ c. steamed rice (1 grain)
½ c. broccoli (1 fruit or vegetable)
1 slice French bread (1 grain)
1 tsp. margarine (1 fat)
½ c. fat-free strawberry frozen yogurt (1 sweet)

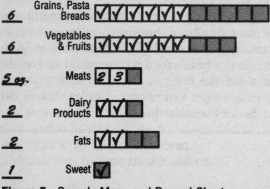

Figure 5. Sample Menu and Record Chart

· 4 ·

MAKING THE SWITCH TO LOW-FAT COOKING

Switching to low-fat cooking doesn't have to be difficult. In fact, it's likely that low-fat cooking won't be any more difficult or time-consuming than the way you already cook.

The recipes in this book were designed with real people in mind. They were meant for the busy homemaker who cooks daily as well as the single adult who rarely cooks more than one or two meals a week. They were developed for people who want to eat healthfully but who also want their food to taste good and to add pleasure to their lives.

Read through the tips in this chapter. There are general tips for lowering the fat in your cooking and eating as well as a section about how to revise your family's favorite recipes. You should be able to find some hints to help you on your path toward healthier eating.

• Determine your fat goal (see Figure 6, below) and make food choices that will allow you to accomplish

FAT ALLOWANCES IN GRAMS

Daily caloric intake	30% calories from fat	20% calories from fat
1200	40	27
1500	50	33
1800	60	40
2100	70	47
2500	83	56

Figure 6. Maximum Daily Fat Allowance

that goal. If you need to include some of your higher-fat favorites to keep from feeling deprived, that's fine; just be extra careful to balance the splurge with low-fat selections at other meals.

• Invest in good nonstick cookware. Cooking in non-stick pans really does reduce the amount of fat needed in preparing foods. To make your new cookware last longer, read and follow manufacturer's instructions for care and cleaning. If you have some favorite older pans, keep them well seasoned. After cleaning, wipe the cooking surface with approximately 2 tsp. oil, and let the pan rest until you use it again.

• Learn new sautéing methods. With good nonstick cookware and nonstick sprays, you won't need to use oil in most cases. "Sweat" your foods by adding a bit of water or broth to the pan instead of fat. If you want your food to brown, cook it until all of the liquid has evaporated, and continue to heat it for a few moments longer; most foods will brown some just from the heat and the natural sugars in the foods.

Some foods don't need to be sautéed at all; they can just cook in the food's juices. For instance, when you make chili, instead of sautéing the onions and green peppers in oil and then adding the tomatoes, add the tomatoes first and let the other vegetables cook in their juice.

- Read labels and nutrition information. Since different brands of the same product can vary widely in their nutritional content, use the information listed on individual labels whenever possible. Read the fat grams as well as the fiber, vitamin, and mineral content when applicable, and pick the product that is best for you.

- Buy and eat more fresh produce, and remember that produce tastes best when it is in season. Many times, fresh produce tastes so much better that you won't need the fat, salt, and sugar that you need for canned and frozen foods. Resort to canned fruits and vegetables only when your favorite ones aren't in season and when you are too rushed to shop for and prepare the fresh.

- Remove all visible fat and skin from meats, chicken, and fish before cooking. Also skim off all fat from meat juices and stocks before making soups and sauces.

- When you do add fat, use fats with a lot of flavor such as extra-virgin olive oil and toasted sesame oil.

- Consider eating more meatless meals. Research has shown that we don't need nearly as much protein as most of us consume, so we can feel safe about leaving the meat out at some meals during the week. Don't worry, either, about complementing proteins; we now know that our bodies can build proteins from amino acids, the building blocks of protein, consumed all during the day. They don't all have to be eaten together at the same meal.

- Use fat-free or low-fat cheese, or use half as much of a strongly flavored cheese such as extra-sharp cheddar or Romano. Since most low-fat cheeses contain half as much fat as their regular counterparts, half of the volume of a regular cheese contains the same fat as the full amount of a low-fat variety. Sometimes, depending on the variety and brand, the smaller amount of the regular cheese has more flavor. Use cheese where it will count the most—often that means sprinkling it on top of the food.

- Boost your fiber intake by using whole wheat bread (100 percent whole wheat is best) instead of white bread whenever possible. Substitute whole wheat flour for half of the white flour in recipes. Keep unprocessed bran on hand, and add some to your breads and cooked cereals; some people like bran sprinkled over cold cereal and salad.

- Go ahead and use your favorite boxed mixes such as Kraft macaroni and cheese, Lipton rice and pasta products, Hungry Jack scalloped potato mixes, and Rice-A-Roni, but make sure the sodium content is not too high for you. They can all be prepared without adding the fat called for. If you do not add the extra fat, the fat content will remain the same as what's listed under "as packaged," not under "as prepared."

- Experiment with new grains. Grains on their own are virtually fat free and are high in healthful complex carbohydrates and fiber. Try substituting brown rice for white in your recipes; just allow for a longer cooking time. Buy some barley, grits, couscous,

Low-Fat Substitutes

INGREDIENTS	SUBSTITUTES
Whole eggs	Egg substitutes such as Egg Beaters, or two egg whites for each egg
Whole milk	Low-fat or skim milk
Cream	Evaporated skim milk, nonfat plain yogurt, fat-free sour cream
Cheese	Fat-free cheese, low-fat cheese, or half as much regular cheese
Cream cheese	Light cream cheese, or Neufchâtel, fat-free cream cheese, or yogurt cheese
Luncheon meats	Very lean ham and turkey breast
Ground beef	Extra-lean ground beef or turkey, or half as much in a casserole or sauce
Butter, margarine	Diet tub margarine, jam, fruit butter, and jelly
Salad dressings	Fat-free or low-fat varieties, balsamic vinegar, lemon juice, salsa, fat-free sour cream with garlic or herbs
Sour cream	Plain nonfat yogurt, fat-free sour cream
Snack foods	Low-fat or fat-free versions, pretzels, rice cakes, air-popped popcorn

bulgur wheat, and millet, and try using them where you might normally use rice or pasta.
• Refer to the list of substitutes above when you shop and cook. Just using these lower fat or fat-free substitutes can cut the fat content of some foods in half—or more!

When trying any fat-free version of a prepared food, try two or three different brands before deciding that you don't like the product, as some brands will taste much better to you than others. If you can't find a nonfat product that you like, use a low-fat version for now, but try fat-free versions again in six months or a year, as food manufacturers keep testing and improving their products.

Revising Your Favorite Recipes

You can continue to use most of your favorite recipes if you're willing to make some changes. If the simple substitutions listed above aren't quite enough, try some of the ideas below. Remember that many recipes can stand a cut in fat up to 50 percent without losing much of the flavor that makes the recipe so special. Experiment until you find the changes that work best for your family's specialties. Even if it takes several trials, the revised recipe will definitely be worth the effort, and you'll enjoy fat and calorie savings for years to come!

MAIN DISHES

Look at your fat sources—meat, butter, margarine, oil, shortening, and cheese. Do you need all of these ingredients? Try omitting the ones that might not be necessary, or reduce the amount you use.

Use fat-free or light sour cream, canned soup, and mayonnaise in place of the older higher-fat versions. Reduce the amount of cheese by half, or use fat-free or low-fat cheese. When a recipe calls for meat or cheese with rice, vegetables, or pasta, cut back on the amount of meat or cheese and boost the amount of the other ingredients. When using meat, buy the leanest cuts and remove all visible skin and fat before cooking.

In many instances, it is possible to eliminate fat altogether when sautéing. Either spray your pan with Pam, or cook the food in a small amount of water or broth instead of fat. Start with ¼ to ½ c. liquid, and add more if needed. Be sure that the liquid evaporates by the end of the cooking period, unless you want some left behind for a sauce.

VEGETABLES AND SALADS

Remember that the main function of fat in vegetable cookery is for sautéing and for adding flavor. Sauté your vegetables in liquid (see above), or reduce the oil to the smallest amount possible. Start with ½ or 1 Tbsp. for most recipes.

For extra flavor, take advantage of the widely available herb seasonings and seasoned salts as well as fat-free bouillon or broth, vinegar, mustard, and ketchup. Experiment with your own seasonings—lemon juice and brown sugar, low-fat or fat-free salad dressing, or fat-free sour cream. Remember to mix colors and add colorful garnishes such as pimiento strips.

BAKED GOODS AND DESSERTS

Fat serves three major functions in baked goods and desserts: flavoring, moisturizing, and tenderizing.

Take advantage of other high-flavor ingredients such as fruits; caraway seeds; vanilla, rum, lemon, or orange extracts; and fruit juices. When nuts are called for, toast them until they're slightly brown and aromatic, and you'll get almost twice the nutty flavor for the same volume of nuts.

Use low-fat or fat-free frosting. Sugar glazes can be made with just powdered sugar and liquid (water, lemon juice, or orange juice), flavor extracts, and spices. Add cocoa powder for a chocolate glaze. Fruit sauces are especially good over low-fat cakes, as they add moisture. Some cakes need no more than a powdered sugar topping or a dollop of Lite Cool Whip.

To provide the moisture that fat usually adds, try substituting pureed fruit or vegetables for all or part of the oil, butter, margarine, or shortening in your cake or bread recipes. A general rule of thumb is one to two times as much fruit as fat, depending on the consistency of the fruit. In darker-colored baked goods, substitute molasses for part of the sugar in a recipe. Keep in mind that batter low in fat will usually be a little bit "wetter" than a fat-based batter.

To keep baked goods tender, take care not to develop the gluten in doughs and batters. In general, do *not* beat the dough after adding flour; stir the flour in gently just until it is all combined. Use cake and pastry flour (a softer wheat flour lower in protein) in cakes, muffins, and sweet breads.

Fat is essential for tenderizing traditional piecrust. Try baking a one-crust pie and garnishing it with fruit or Lite Cool Whip. Or substitute a crumb crust made with just enough fat to hold it in shape. Sometimes you can turn your pie into a different type of dessert while still retaining the flavor that makes it so special to you. For example, consider baking an apple crisp instead of apple pie, a pumpkin cake in place of pumpkin pie, or mincemeat bread pudding rather than a traditional mincemeat pie.

Whenever possible, decrease the number of eggs, or use two egg whites rather than one whole egg—or use fat-free egg substitutes such as Egg Beaters. For full-sized cakes, two whole eggs is generally enough. If you omit eggs entirely, you may find it necessary to add 2 to 4 Tbsp. water for each egg omitted. You may also need to add a bit more baking powder or baking soda. And, as with all recipes, substitute skim milk for whole milk or cream.

Reading Labels

Food manufacturers are giving us more information than ever to aid us in making wiser decisions about the foods we buy. But sometimes manufacturers tell us more than we need, and some of the information is misleading. For instance, "95 percent fat-free" seems to mean "low in fat," but it's possible that *all* of the product's calories come from fat—if the food is 95 percent water.

The new stricter nutritional labeling regulations should help consumers, but don't expect the manufacturer to make your decisions for you. Instead, learn now how to arm yourself in a marketplace where the bottom line is selling, not necessarily providing healthful foods.

Tips for Understanding Labeling Data

1. Remember that a food's package is the company's last chance to get a consumer to buy the product. So don't focus on the front of the package. Instead, go straight to the nutritional label on the *back* of the package.

2. Find the number of fat grams. Know your goal for the day, and decide whether this product will fit into your goals. Compare this number with that of competing products—there's sometimes a large difference between brands. Blindfold taste tests have shown that sometimes the foods with less fat taste just as good as—or even better than—the higher fat products.

3. Don't pay extra for foods that are marked "low-fat" when the food itself is generally low-fat anyway—for example, sliced turkey breast.

4. Don't be fooled by the terms like "low-fat," "low-calorie," or "light." These terms simply mean that the foods contain fewer calories or less fat than the original. While that's an improvement, these foods may still provide more fat and calories than you want.

5. Don't rely too heavily on "% calories from fat." While this is a helpful guide for setting overall goals, it isn't always useful when selecting individual foods. Remember that the percentage is a relationship between the number of fat calories and the total number of calories. Because of this, it is possible for the manufacturer to lower that percentage—and make the product *seem* more desirable—by increasing the number of total calories—in other words, by increasing sugar calories. Some muffins, for example, have a lower percentage of calories from fat because they are

higher in sugar, but their labels show that they contain the same amount of fat.

Some foods such as tub margarine derive 100 percent of their calories from fat, but you can still use them in small amounts, especially with fat-free or very low-fat foods. So always keep your fat goal in mind, and be aware of fat grams.

6. Take note of the fiber content listed on the label. Sometimes in our obsession with fat we forget that fiber's very important too.

7. Check *all* of the nutritional information on the label. Just because a food has one nutritional virtue— low sugar content, for example—don't assume it is healthful in all ways. One brand-name ice cream bar, for instance, is sugar-free, but each bar contains 11 grams of fat. At 140 calories per bar, that means 70 percent of the calories come from fat.

8. Don't be overwhelmed by all of the information provided on the label. Once you learn to read labels critically, you'll be able to find the information you want quickly and ignore the rest.

Time Savers for Healthful Cooking

If you are new to low-fat cooking, you're probably concerned about how much time these new changes are going to add to your already busy schedule.

There are steps that you can take to ensure that preparing healthful low-fat meals is no more time-consuming than cooking your higher-fat fare. The tips below will help you when you just don't have time to spend in the kitchen or when there are other things you'd rather do with your time.

1. *Shop wisely*. Get into the habit of reading labels, especially when you buy frozen or processed foods. Pay no attention to claims like "93% fat-free," since they can be misleading. Look for the actual fat content in grams, or note the percentage of calories from fat.

Buy lean meats without much marbling (streaks of fat throughout the meat). Purchase skim or nonfat dairy products such as fat-free sour cream, cottage cheese, and yogurt. Buy frozen vegetables without sauce, as most sauces contain fats. If you eat meat, always keep some boneless lean meat and poultry in the freezer for quick meals.

2. *Learn low-fat cooking techniques and use them regularly*. Once you know them well, you'll find that it doesn't take any more time to cook with a small amount of fat than with lots of it. Learn to sauté in broth or water instead of oil. When you do use fat choose a flavorful one such as extra-virgin or first-press olive oil or one of Joyce Chen's Oriental stir-fry oils.

3. *If your schedule doesn't allow you to cook every day, try to cook at least three times each week—but prepare double portions*. This way, you'll always have leftovers. Either reheat them and serve them as they were the first day, or vary them by adding a sauce or mixing them with pasta.

4. *Remember that a little bit of planning helps save time later*. Make complete grocery lists to avoid extra trips to the store. When you return from the store, wash and cut up some of your vegetables and seal them in sealable plastic bags so that you are always ready for a stir-fry in a moment's notice. Boning chicken before freezing it means that you'll always be only thirty minutes away from a chicken skillet dinner of fajitas.

5. *Start a file of fast recipes.* Most of us file recipes by categorizing them into entrées, casseroles, soups, breads, and desserts. But why not have a separate file just for fast recipes? It will save the time of flipping through lots of recipes.

Make your file more efficient by tossing out those recipes you've clipped from magazines and newspapers but aren't really going to use. If you haven't used a few recipes that you think you really want, put them aside to try this week. If they're not special enough to try the first week, then you'll probably never use them. Throw them away.

6. *Reorganize your cupboards every six months.* Spending thirty minutes to an hour can save time later by making it easier for you to find what you need. When you reorganize, put aside all the foods you don't use anymore—fatty foods left over from your less healthy days, and foods that are no longer fresh. Some research has shown that rancid fats may injure the arterial wall, giving plaque a place to start building up. Rancid fats can be found in boxed foods past their expiration date. If you're accustomed to fresh food, some boxed foods may taste stale or soapy to you—a sign of rancid fats.

KEEP THESE FOODS ON HAND FOR FAST MEALS

FROZEN MEATS AND ENTRÉES: Low-fat frozen dinners or homemade meals prepared from leftovers. Frozen kits for fajitas or stir-fries (omit the oil).

MEATS: Frozen turkey steaks or very lean beef or pork

steaks for stir-fries. Boneless chicken breast and fish squares.

GRAINS, RICE, AND BEANS: Uncooked rice and pasta. Refrigerated cooked rice and pasta. Canned beans. Boxed or packaged rice and pasta mixes (omit fats and use skim milk).

QUICK SAUCES: Fat-free sour cream, yogurt, salsa, and barbecue sauce to combine with noodles or rice or add to chicken or fish.

VEGETABLES: Fresh, frozen, and canned vegetables. Crushed tomatoes for easy tomato sauce (heat tomato with basil, oregano, garlic, onion; serve over pasta or chicken).

FRUITS: Many varieties of canned, fresh, and frozen fruits.

BREADS: Refrigerated biscuit dough with low fat content. Frozen bread dough.

DESSERTS: Instant puddings (use skim milk), gelatin desserts, light cake and brownie mixes with low fat content. Fat-free yogurt, frozen yogurt, light frozen dairy desserts, sherbet.

SNACKS: Light popcorn, fat-free crackers, pretzels, gingersnaps, graham crackers, Fig Newtons, cereal, low-fat snack foods.

LOW-FAT MENUS FOR
SPECIAL OCCASIONS

---◆---

FALL AND WINTER MENUS

Thanksgiving or Christmas Day Dinner

MARINATED TURKEY BREAST WITH ORANGE GLAZE
(p. 85)
SAVORY BREAD STUFFING (p. 161)
SPICED SWEET POTATO SLICES (p. 159)
LEMONY GREEN BEANS (p. 149)
FRUITED CRANBERRY SALAD (p. 175)
OLD-FASHIONED DINNER ROLLS (p. 186)
PUMPKIN CAKE WITH ALMOND GLAZE (p. 227)

**One serving of each food listed = 560 calories, 5.4 g fat,
8.7% calories from fat**

Winter Dinner Party #1

POTATO-SCALLION SOUP (p. 80)
POACHED SALMON SQUARES (p. 103)
RICE
STEAMED FRESH BROCCOLI
OLD-FASHIONED DINNER ROLLS (p. 186)
APPLE BUNDLES (p. 255)

> One serving of each food listed = 726 calories, 8.6 g fat,
> 10.7% calories from fat

Winter Dinner Party #2

PEPPERED HERB CHEESE BALL (p. 56)
CREAMY MUSHROOM SOUP (p. 75)
HAM STEAK WITH CRANBERRY SAUCE (p. 113)
ROASTED POTATO WEDGES (p. 158)
LEMONY GREEN BEANS (p. 149)
FRENCH BREAD (p. 183)
COCOA ANGEL ROLL (p. 237)

> One serving of each food listed = 765 calories, 10.6 g
> fat, 12.5% calories from fat

After-Work Dinner Party

FRESH FRUIT CUP
HONEY-MUSTARD PORK MEDALLIONS (p. 114)
BOILED POTATOES
LETTUCE AND ORANGE SALAD (p. 170)

WHITE BEER BREAD (p. 195)
CHOCOLATE BELGIAN WAFFLES (p. 260)

> One serving of each food listed = 786 calories, 12.5 g fat, 14.3% calories from fat

Quick Super Bowl Chili Party

FAT-FREE GUACAMOLE AND BAKED TORTILLA CHIPS
  (p. 60)
SPICY TURKEY CHILI (p. 88)
TOSSED ROMAINE SALAD WITH CROUTONS
  (p. 168–69)
FRENCH BREAD (p. 183)
MOIST CHOCOLATE CAKE WITH CHOCOLATE
  FROSTING (p. 223–24)

> One serving of each food listed = 627 calories, 8.3 g fat, 11.9% calories from fat

Simple Midwinter's Night Stew-Pot

HEARTY BEEF STEW (p. 109)
LETTUCE SALAD WITH FAT-FREE GARLIC-
  PEPPERCORN DRESSING (p. 287)
WHITE BEER BREAD (p. 195)
GINGERBREAD WITH LEMON SAUCE (p. 232)

> One serving of each food listed = 486 calories, 4.4 g fat, 8.1% calories from fat

SPRING AND SUMMER MENUS

Summer Luncheon Buffet

SALMON MOUSSE (p. 54) WITH FAT-FREE WHEAT
    CRACKERS
ORIENTAL CHICKEN SALAD (p. 96)
PINEAPPLE FRUIT BOWL (p. 174)
FRENCH BREAD (p. 183)
LEMON MERINGUE PIE (p. 258)

> One serving of each food listed = 665 calories, 10.6 g
> fat, 14.3% calories from fat

Cookout No. 1

MARINATED SEAFOOD KEBABS (p. 105)
STEAMED RICE
ZUCCHINI FANS (p. 154)
TOMATO WEDGES WITH SWEET BASIL VINAIGRETTE
    (p. 171)
FRENCH BREAD (p. 183)
APRICOT CREAM CAKE (p. 240)

> One serving of each food listed = 502 calories, 4.3 g fat,
> 7.7% calories from fat

Cookout No. 2

TANDOORI CHICKEN (p. 93)
INDIAN POTATOES (p. 157)

CUCUMBER-YOGURT SALAD (p. 172)
PITA BREAD
CREAMY CHEESECAKE (p. 243) WITH FRESH
    RASPBERRIES

> One serving of each food listed = 555 calories, 8.4 g fat,
> 13.6% calories from fat

Weekend Brunch

PASTA SALAD (p. 179)
FRUIT KEBABS (p. 273)
ASSORTED MUFFINS (p. 204)
ICE CREAM CAKE (p. 239)

> One serving of each food listed = 463 calories, 3.1 g fat,
> 6.0% calories from fat

Southern Summer Meal

CRISPY OVEN-"FRIED" CHICKEN (p. 87)
ALL-AMERICAN MACARONI AND CHEESE (p. 131)
TOMATO WEDGES WITH SWEET BASIL VINAIGRETTE
    (p. 171)
DROP BISCUITS (p. 194)
FRESH PEACH COBBLER (p. 257)

> One serving of each food listed = 476 calories, 6.5 g fat,
> 12.3% calories from fat

ETHNIC MENUS

Indian Curry

CHICKEN-YOGURT CURRY (p. 94)
STEAMED BASMATI RICE
CUCUMBER-YOGURT SALAD (p. 172)
TOMATO CHUTNEY (p. 276)
PITA BREAD
OLD-FASHIONED "ICE CREAM" FLOATS (p. 275)

> One serving of each food listed = 428 calories, 3.4 g fat, 7.1% calories from fat

East Asian Dinner

QUICK AND EASY HOT AND SOUR SOUP (p. 74)
BEEF AND BROCCOLI WITH PEANUT SAUCE (p. 111)
STEAMED RICE
OLD-FASHIONED DINNER ROLLS
FROZEN FRUIT SALAD (p. 265)

> One serving of each food listed = 492 calories, 8.6 g fat, 15.7% calories from fat

Italian Dinner

CHICKEN MARSALA (p. 92)
PASTA WITH "CREAM SAUCE" (p. 118)—half-serving as side dish
TOSSED ROMAINE SALAD (p. 168) WITH OLIVE OIL DRESSING

FRENCH BREAD (p. 183)
CREAMY CHEESECAKE TOPPED WITH FRESH RED
 RASPBERRIES (p. 243)

> One serving of each food listed = 602 calories, 12.4 g
> fat, 18.5% calories from fat

Mexican Dinner

MEXICAN BEAN DIP (p. 55) WITH BAKED TORTILLA
 CHIPS
CHEESE ENCHILADAS WITH RED CHILI SAUCE (p. 135)
MEXICAN RICE (p. 160)
SHREDDED TOMATO, LETTUCE, AND ONION
SOUTHWESTERN CORN MUFFINS (p. 217)
LOW-FAT HOT CHOCOLATE SPRINKLED WITH
 GROUND CINNAMON (p. 61)

> One serving of each food listed = 755 calories, 13.2 g
> fat, 15.7% calories from fat

APPETIZERS
AND
BEVERAGES

———◆———

When I first started eating healthfully, I stopped serving appetizers altogether. It seemed that all of our favorite appetizers were laden with cheese, sour cream, cream cheese, and other fatty foods, and I felt utterly deprived settling for vegetables or fruit with cottage cheese or yogurt-based dips.

Here are some new ideas for appetizers that are tasty but also low in the fat-filled ingredients that you want to avoid. Remember that they all seem to taste even better when beautifully arranged on plates or platters with colorful accompaniments like lettuce and fresh fruits, and when served with tasty fat-free beverages like those included in this section.

Salmon Mousse

◆

Consider buying a fish mold if you plan to make this often, as the fish shape makes an elegant presentation. I always use fresh salmon for special occasions, but canned salmon is also very good. Chicken of the Sea markets skinless and boneless canned salmon, if you can find it. If not, use another brand low in fat. Try serving leftover mousse on pita bread with tomato slices and shredded lettuce. It's a treat!

1 can (10¾ oz.) Campbell's Healthy Request cream of
    mushroom soup
1 envelope unflavored gelatin
¾ c. finely chopped celery
¼ c. finely chopped onion
2 Tbsp. minced fresh parsley, or 2 tsp. parsley flakes
1 Tbsp. fresh lemon juice
1 salmon steak (approx. 10 oz.), poached and flaked,
    bone and skin discarded, or 1 can (6⅛ oz.) pink
    salmon
1 c. fat-free sour cream

Lightly coat 4-cup mold with vegetable oil spray. Pour soup into saucepan. Add gelatin and bring to a boil, stirring constantly. Remove from heat, and add remaining ingredients except sour cream. When well combined, stir in sour cream until well mixed. Pour mixture into mold. Refrigerate at least 3 hours, or until well set.

To serve, loosen slightly by inserting knife carefully between mousse and pan in a few places. Then invert mousse onto serving plate and serve with fat-free or low-fat crackers.

YIELD: 3¼ c.

Each ¼ c. serving (without crackers): 44 calories, 0.8 g fat (15.7% calories from fat), 0.4 g saturated fat, 0.4 g polyunsaturated fat, <0.1 g monounsaturated fat, 6 mg cholesterol, 4.4 g carbohydrate, 5.2 g protein, 216 mg sodium

EXCHANGES: 1 vegetable; ½ lean meat

Mexican Bean Dip

———◆———

Serve this dip hot or cold with baked tortilla chips or chunks of pita bread, or use it as a topping for a nacho plate. Use it, too, to create a meatless pita sandwich with alfalfa sprouts and other raw chopped vegetables.

1 can (16 oz.) black beans, drained (reserve juice), or 2
    c. cooked black beans (from dried)
1 clove garlic
2 Tbsp. onion

Place beans in food processor or blender along with garlic and onion. Process, adding just enough reserved juice so that the mixture will process and become smooth. (If you are using your own cooked black beans, you may not need extra liquid. If you do, use water.)

To serve warm, place in bowl and microwave until hot, stirring midway through cooking period, or heat in saucepan, replacing liquid if necessary.

YIELD: approx. 2 c.

Each 2 Tbsp. serving: 29 calories, 0.1 g fat (3.1% calories

from fat), <0.1 g saturated fat, <0.1 g polyunsaturated fat, <0.1 g monounsaturated fat, 0 mg cholesterol, 5.2 g carbohydrate, 1.9 g protein, 70 mg sodium (Sodium content will be lower with home-cooked beans.)

EXCHANGES: ½ bread

Peppered Herb Cheese Ball

━━━◆━━━

Here is a soft fat-free cheese that you can make yourself. Look for cheesecloth in specialty kitchen stores, some supermarkets, and hardware stores. Even though the process takes several hours, you spend only a few minutes in actual preparation.

    1 qt. nonfat plain yogurt
    ½ clove garlic, pressed
    2 Tbsp. finely minced onion
    2 Tbsp. finely chopped fresh parsley, or 2 tsp. parsley
        flakes
    ¼ tsp. salt
    ⅛ tsp. ground black pepper
    Optional: Other favorite herbs

Line a large bowl with two layers of cheesecloth. Each strip of cheesecloth should be about 2 feet long and hang evenly over each side of the bowl. Scoop yogurt into center of cheesecloth, pull edges of cloth up over yogurt to form a bundle, and lift bundle out of bowl. Tie longer ends of cheesecloth over a water faucet so that the bundle of yogurt hangs from the faucet. Leave for 5 to 6 hours or overnight. Liquid will drip from the yogurt, leaving approximately one cup of cheese the consistency of cream cheese.

Mix remaining ingredients into cheese, wrap mixture in plastic wrap, and shape into a ball. Store in refrigerator. Serve as a cheese spread with fat-free or low-fat crackers.

YIELD: one ball (approx. 1 c.)

Each 1 Tbsp. serving: 33 calories, 0.1 g fat (2.7% calories from fat), <0.1 g saturated fat, <0.1 g polyunsaturated fat, <0.1 g monounsaturated fat, 0 mg cholesterol, 4.6 g carbohydrate, 3.3 g protein, 78 mg sodium

EXCHANGES: ½ skim milk

Dipping Sauce for Bread Sticks

————◆————

Use this recipe as a dip for breadsticks, as a spread for French or Italian bread, or as a red sauce for your pasta dishes. Not only is it flavorful and low-fat, but it's also quick and easy.

3 cloves garlic, pressed
1 medium onion, chopped
1 Tbsp. olive oil
Optional: ½ tsp. crushed red pepper
1 can (28 oz.) crushed tomatoes with puree
1 can (5 oz.) tomato paste plus 1 can water
1 tsp. dried basil
½ tsp. dried oregano
Optional: ½ tsp. salt

Sauté garlic and onion in olive oil until tender, about 5 minutes. Add red pepper, if desired, along with remaining ingredients. Heat to boiling (watch for popping), and immediately reduce heat to low-medium. Cook 15 minutes, or until flavors are blended.

YIELD: 5c.

Each ¼ c. serving: 31 calories, 0.8 g fat (23% calories from fat), 0.1 g saturated fat, 1.1 g polyunsaturated fat, 0.5 g monounsaturated fat, 0 mg cholesterol, 6.1 g carbohydrate, 1.1 g protein, 13 mg sodium

EXCHANGES: 1 vegetable

Salsa

———◆———

Commercial salsa can be quite expensive compared to home-made. Next time you want salsa, try making your own using this recipe. It will taste best if you allow it to sit in the refrigerator for two or three days before you serve it, so, when time allows, make the salsa ahead of time.

  2 cans (14½ oz. each) whole peeled tomatoes, well
     drained
  1 clove garlic
  1 small onion, chopped
  ½ tsp. chopped cilantro leaves
  ⅛ tsp. salt
  ⅛ tsp. ground black pepper
  1 tsp. minced jalapeño peppers, or more, to taste

Chop well-drained tomatoes with whisk. Add remaining ingredients and mix well. Taste and add more chopped jalapeño peppers, if you wish. Refrigerate mixture until ready to use.

YIELD: 2c.

Each 2 Tbsp. serving: 8 calories, 0 g fat (0% calories from fat), 0 g saturated fat, 0 g polyunsaturated fat, 0 g monounsaturated fat, 0 mg cholesterol, 1.7 g carbohydrate, 0.3 g protein, 59 mg sodium

EXCHANGES: ⅓ vegetable

Chipotle Salsa

———◆———

This recipe was inspired by a recipe from *Salsa* by P. J. Birosik. In this version, I've left out all added fat and made use of ingredients I can readily find. The chipotle peppers give this mixture a pleasant smoky flavor that's quite different from other salsas. It's great for dipping as well as for topping rice, burritos, and other Mexican foods. If your supermarket doesn't sell chipotle peppers, look for them in a Latin American or specialty food store.

1 can (28 oz.) tomatillos, drained
1 can (16 oz.) canned whole tomatoes, drained
Slightly less than half of a 7.5 oz. can chipotle peppers,
    with juice
4 cloves garlic
¼ c. packed cilantro leaves

Blend or process all ingredients together until only a few small chunks remain. Pour mixture into ungreased hot skillet, cover skillet loosely to prevent spattering, and boil salsa until thickened.

Serve warm or cold with chips, or over rice or fish.

YIELD: approx. 2 cups

Each 2 Tbsp. serving: 18 calories, 0.4 g fat (19.2% calories from fat). <0.1 g saturated fat, <0.1 g polyunsaturated fat, <0.1 g monounsaturated fat, 0 mg cholesterol, 3.7 g carbohydrate, 0.1 g protein, 148 mg sodium

EXCHANGES: 1 vegetable

Fat-Free Guacamole

———◆———

If you're like me, you loved guacamole until you found out how much fat it contains. Its main ingredient is mashed avocado, which averages a whopping 38 grams of fat per cup!

Here is an alternative made with fat-free asparagus. If you're a guacamole fan, this is definitely worth a try. We've enjoyed it.

    1 can (14½ oz.) asparagus, drained
    2 tsp. lime juice
    2 Tbsp. finely chopped onion
    2 cloves pressed garlic
    2 Tbsp. chopped tomatoes or sweet red pepper
    ⅛ tsp. cayenne
    1½ Tbsp. chopped fresh cilantro leaves, or ½ tsp. dried
        cilantro (coriander)
    Optional: Pinch salt and black pepper

Mash or coarsely process asparagus until it is almost pureed, but still contains some small chunks. Add remaining ingredients, cover, and refrigerate for several hours before use.

YIELD: approx. 2 c.

Each 2 Tbsp. serving: 6 calories, 0 g fat (0% calories from fat), 0 g saturated fat, 0 g polyunsaturated fat, 0 g monounsaturated fat, 0 mg cholesterol, 1.1 g carbohydrate, 0.6 g protein, 50 mg sodium

EXCHANGES: Free

Low-Fat Hot Chocolate

———◆———

Ever since I began making this recipe, my family hasn't wanted any more hot chocolate mixes. This hot chocolate recipe is hardly any more work than the instant variety, and it is always made fresh without the dried skim milk flavor of packaged mixes. For a delightful change, try the suggested variations below.

1 Tbsp. cocoa powder
1–1½ Tbsp. sugar or sugar substitute
1 mug skim milk (measure in mug)
¼ tsp. vanilla extract

Stir cocoa powder and sugar together in heavy saucepan until most of the lumps are gone. Add milk, and heat to a simmer (do not boil), stirring constantly and mashing out any clumps of chocolate against side of pan with back of spoon. Remove from heat and add vanilla extract. Stir in one of the ingredients below, if desired.

YIELD: 1 mug hot chocolate

Each 1 cup serving: 177 calories, 1.3 g fat (6.8% calories from fat), 0.4 g saturated fat, 0.0 g polyunsaturated fat, 0.1 g

monounsaturated fat, 5 mg cholesterol, 29.3 g carbohydrate, 11.8 g protein, 160 mg sodium

EXCHANGES: 1 skim milk; 1 fruit

VARIATIONS: Add one of the following ingredients to each mug.

marshmallow, or 1 dollop Lite Cool Whip
1 tsp. instant coffee granules
1 Tbsp. amaretto (almond) liqueur
2 Tbsp. Frangelico (hazelnut) liqueur
2 Tbsp. Grand Marnier, or 1 Tbsp. curaçao (orange liqueur)
1 tsp. creme de menthe

Minted Tea

Nothing beats a glass of mint-flavored tea on a hot summer's day. If you don't already have it, you may want to consider planting some mint in your yard to brew a pitcher at a moment's notice. To prevent the mint from spreading throughout your flower bed, consider planting it in a large pot or window box.

1 qt. boiling water
6–8 tea bags (regular or decaffeinated)
6–10 fresh mint leaves
1 qt. cold water

Pour boiling water over tea bags and mint leaves in 2-qt. pitcher. Let mixture steep for 10 minutes, and then remove tea bags and mint. (For a stronger mint flavor, leave mint in tea.) Add cold water, stir well, and serve over ice.

Y I E L D : 2 qt.

Each 8 oz. serving: 2 calories, 0 g fat (0% calories from fat), 0 g saturated fat, 0 g polyunsaturated fat, 0 g monounsaturated fat, 0 mg cholesterol, <1 g carbohydrate, 0 g protein, 0 mg sodium

E X C H A N G E S : free

Fruited Teas

————◆————

Fruit-flavored teas have become very popular, but there's no need to buy them. Here's a recipe for an affordable tea that you can make at home. Use any fruit juice you like. The berry flavors are my favorite.

If you want to save calories, use a juice concentrate sweetened with aspartame (NutraSweet) instead of sugar.

½ c. frozen fruit juice concentrate, thawed
1 qt. brewed tea

Stir the juice concentrate into the pitcher of tea, and serve over ice.

Y I E L D : approx. 4 c.

Each 8 oz. serving: 67 calories, 0.1 g fat (1.3% calories from fat), <0.1 g saturated fat, <0.1 g polyunsaturated fat, <0.1 g monounsaturated fat, 0 mg cholesterol, 16.5 g carbohydrate, 0.2 g protein, 8 mg sodium

E X C H A N G E S : 1 fruit

Fruit Sparklers

——◆——

Sparklers are an easy alternative to soda, and they're less expensive than bottled flavored water. Serve them at your next get-together for your guests who prefer a nonalcoholic drink. Grape and cranberry sparklers are two of my favorites.

   1 qt. cold fruit juice
   1 qt. cold club soda

Mix juice and club soda just before serving. Serve over ice.

YIELD: 2 qt.

Each 8 oz. serving with cranberry juice: 72 calories, 0 g fat (0% calories from fat), 0 g saturated fat, 0 g polyunsaturated fat, 0 g monounsaturated fat, 0 mg cholesterol, 18 g carbohydrate, 0 g protein, 28 mg sodium

EXCHANGES: 1 fruit

Each 8 oz. serving with low-calorie cranberry juice cocktail: 22 calories, 0 g fat (0% calories from fat), 0 g saturated fat, 0 g polyunsaturated fat, 0 g monounsaturated fat, 0 mg cholesterol, 5.5 g carbohydrate, 0 g protein, 29 mg sodium

EXCHANGES: ⅓ fruit

Mulled Cider

——◆——

Nothing's better than a cup of hot cider on a cold night; your whole house will smell wonderful while the beverage mulls in an open pot. Add more spices, if you like a spicier cider. I usually leave in a few of the oranges and cinnamon sticks if I'm serving the mulled drink in a bowl. If you make more than you can drink, refrigerate the cider, and reheat it on top of the stove or in the microwave.

1 gallon apple cider or apple juice
4 cinnamon sticks, broken in half
10–15 whole cloves
10–15 whole allspice
2 oranges, quartered

Place all ingredients in large pot, and bring mixture to a boil. Reduce heat, cover, and simmer 30 minutes to 1 hour, until spicy and ready to serve. Remove spices with slotted spoon, or strain cider before serving.

YIELD: approx. 1 gal.

Each 8 oz. serving: 116 calories, 0.3 g fat (2.3% calories from fat), 0 g saturated fat, 0.1 g polyunsaturated fat, 0 g monounsaturated fat, 0 mg cholesterol, 29 g carbohydrate, 0.3 g protein, 7 mg sodium

EXCHANGES: 2 fruits

Soups

◆

I still remember the day I decided to make my first pot of homemade soup. My mother had made soup once or twice a week during the winter when I was little. Back then the process had seemed magically impossible to me, since I never saw her make a soup exactly the same way twice. I think it wouldn't have seemed so magical if she had used a recipe, but instead, she quite casually took the leftovers from the refrigerator and added them to her large pot. She supplemented them with vegatables she'd canned and frozen from our summer garden, and then she let the soup cook for hours until it was wonderfully delicious and comforting. I knew that the ease with which she made the soup meant she possessed a special talent that few people had.

Back then I never dreamed I would ever be able to do the same. The day I decided to try making soup myself, I felt no less intimidated than I had as a child. However, I knew I would never learn if I never tried, so I called my mother and asked her how she made her soup. We decided to start with vegetable soup since it had been my favorite, and we came as close as we could to creating a recipe for her soup, adjusting for store-bought can sizes instead of the quart jars and freezer containers that she had used. My soup turned out surprisingly well, but to this day, even though my friends rave about my soup, it still doesn't taste quite as good to me as my mother's did back then.

Here are some soups that you can make, all low in fat but full of good taste. If you've never made soup before, don't be intimidated, as I was with my first attempts. Most people agree that homemade soup is one of the easiest and most rewarding foods to make. Teamed with good bread and a salad or fruit, soup can't be beat, especially on a cold winter day.

Homemade Chicken Stock

Nothing's better than homemade chicken or turkey stock in soups and sauces. Here is a simple recipe that will give you the base for a wonderful homemade soup. Use a whole chicken, if you like, or save up unused chicken parts such as backs and wings in a large zipper bag in the freezer, and use them.

If you have a gravy skimmer or separator (available in most stores where kitchen gadgets are sold), you can save time by defatting stock while it is still warm. The skimmer is designed with a spout which pours from the bottom of the container rather than out of the top. To use the skimmer, pour stock into the skimmer, and let it sit for 5–10 minutes. The broth will separate into two layers—a top layer of fat and a bottom layer of fat-free broth. Pour the lower broth layer into a bowl, stopping when the fat reaches the spout. Discard the fat left in the skimmer.

3–4 lb. chicken or turkey, whole or in pieces
5 c. water
Optional: 1 coarsely chopped large onion, 1 stalk celery
   cut into large chunks, bay leaf or thyme to taste.

Add chicken to water in large pot along with any optional ingredients desired. Cover, and boil until chicken is well cooked. Remove chicken from pot.

Defat the stock by refrigerating it until cold and then removing the solid fat layer from the top, or by using a gravy skimmer.

Use the stock in any recipe that calls for chicken stock or broth. If desired, remove meat from bones and reserve for other uses.

YIELD: **Approx. 4 c. stock**

Each 1 c. serving with no added salt: Approx. 15 calories, 0.3 g fat (18% calories from fat), 0.1 g saturated fat, 0.1 g polyunsaturated fat, 0 g monounsaturated fat, 3 mg cholesterol, 0.7 g carbohydrate, 2.5 g protein, 95 mg sodium

EXCHANGES: **free**

Country Chicken-Rice Soup

This was my grandmother's favorite soup. To this day, I love corn and rice in chicken soup, but since part of my family prefers the Chicken-Noodle soup, I alternate between the two variations. Once you try this, I doubt you'll ever want canned chicken soup again.

5–6 c. homemade chicken stock, or 2 cans (14½ oz. each) chicken broth plus 1 c. water
¾ c. diced celery
½ c. chopped onion or scallions
¼ c. grated carrots

½ c. uncooked rice, or ¼ c. uncooked rice and ¼ c.
   uncooked barley
½ c. frozen corn or drained canned corn
1 c. diced cooked chicken or turkey
1 tsp. salt (¼ tsp. if broth contains salt)
⅛ tsp. ground black pepper

Place chicken broth, celery, onion, carrots, and rice
(or rice and barley) in 4 qt. saucepan. Heat to a rolling
boil, and then reduce heat to a simmer. Cover and
simmer until rice (or rice and barley) are tender,
stirring every 10–15 minutes. Add corn and chicken.
Season with salt and pepper, and adjust to taste.
Serve hot.

YIELD: 10 servings

Each ¾ c. serving: 85 calories, 1.1 g fat (11.6% calories from
fat), 0.3 g saturated fat, 0.2 g polyunsaturated fat, 0.4 g
monounsaturated fat, 18 mg cholesterol, 10 g carbohydrate, 9
g protein, 240 mg sodium

EXCHANGES: 1 extra-lean meat; 1 bread

VARIATION: To prepare Chicken-Noodle Soup, follow the recipe for Country Chicken Rice Soup, above,
but use 2 c. very fine egg noodles in place of the rice,
or rice and barley, and cook the soup only until the
noodles are tender.

YIELD: 10 servings

Each ¾ c. serving: 96 calories, 1.5 g fat (14.1% calories from
fat), 0.3 g saturated fat, 0.2 g polyunsaturated fat, 0.4 g
monounsaturated fat, 18 mg cholesterol, 11 g carbohydrate, 9
g protein, 241 mg sodium

EXCHANGES: 1 extra-lean meat; 1 bread

Mexican Tomato-Bean Soup

◆

Here's a soup that doesn't require a long simmering period. As soon as it is heated thoroughly, it is ready to serve. Use mild picante sauce for a less spicy soup, or choose hot sauce for a spicier flavor. Serve this soup with bread, fruit, and a salad for a complete meal.

1 can (28 oz.) whole tomatoes
2 beef bouillon cubes
½ c. medium picante sauce
1 tsp. ground cumin
1½ tsp. finely chopped fresh cilantro or ¾ tsp. dried
    (coriander)
Juice of ½ small lime
2 cans (16 oz. each) black beans, drained and washed
Optional garnishes: sprig of cilantro, dollop of fat-free
    sour cream

Pour tomatoes into large pot, and mash them with a whisk, leaving a few chunks. Add remaining ingredients, except beans and garnishes, and heat to a boil. Reduce heat, and simmer 5–10 minutes. Add beans and heat through. Ladle into bowls, and garnish with cilantro and sour cream, if desired.

YIELD: 8 servings

Each ¾ c. serving: 111 calories, 0.7 g fat (5.7% calories from fat), 0.2 g saturated fat, 0.3 g polyunsaturated fat, 0.1 g monounsaturated fat, 0 mg cholesterol, 20.7 g carbohydrate, 7.2 g protein, 329 mg sodium

EXCHANGES: 1 bread; 1 vegetable

Beef Barley Soup

◆

This soup tastes very rich and beefy—not at all what you would expect a low-fat soup to taste like. Shop for the leanest beef possible, and cut away all visible fat before adding it to your pot.

1 lb. lean stew beef
4 c. water
1 medium onion, chopped
1 stalk celery, chopped
1 carrot, shredded
1 c. uncooked pearl barley
1 tsp. salt
¼ tsp. ground black pepper
Optional: ½ tsp. dried thyme, crushed

Add beef to water in large pot, and heat to boiling. Reduce heat, cover, and simmer about 30 minutes, or until beef is very tender. Remove beef, refrigerate broth, and when cool, remove fatty layer from top, or use a gravy skimmer.

Chop cooked beef into smaller chunks. Add beef to broth along with onion, celery, carrot, and barley. Bring to a boil, reduce heat, and simmer until barley is cooked (about 45 minutes). Taste, and add salt, pepper, and thyme if desired. If necessary, add water until soup reaches the preferred consistency.

YIELD: 8 servings

Each ¾ c. serving: 179 calories, 3.4 g fat (17.1% calories from fat), 1.1 g saturated fat, 0.1 g polyunsaturated fat, 1.2 g

monounsaturated fat, 37 mg cholesterol, 21.6 g carbohydrate, 20.4 g protein, 304 mg sodium

EXCHANGES: 2 extra-lean meats, 1 bread, 1 vegetable

Creamy Broccoli Soup

—————◆—————

This soup is great for guests or for every day, and it can be made in less than half an hour. For an elegant presentation, I puree it finely, sometimes adding tarragon leaves, and I garnish it as suggested. However, for everyday meals, I like it with small chunks of broccoli still in it.

```
2 c. homemade chicken stock, or 1 can (14½ oz.)
    chicken broth or bouillon
2 c. broccoli florets
1 small onion, cut into 8 wedges
3 Tbsp. cornstarch
1½ c. cold skim milk
Salt and ground black pepper to taste
Optional garnish: fresh or dried tarragon leaves or
    chopped scallions
```

Combine chicken stock, broccoli, and onion in 2–4 quart saucepan. Bring mixture to a boil, cover, and reduce heat. Cook approximately 10 minutes longer, until vegetables are very tender. Pour into bowl of food processor and puree, or chop coarsely if you prefer chunks of broccoli in soup. Pour mixture back into saucepan. Stir cornstarch into cold milk until no lumps remain. Pour milk mixture into broccoli mixture, and heat, stirring constantly, until soup thickens and just begins to boil. Remove from heat, season with salt and pepper, and serve hot, garnished with tarragon or chopped scallions if desired.

YIELD: 6 servings

Each ¾ c. serving (without added salt): 49 calories, 0.3 g fat (4.4% calories from fat), 0.1 g saturated fat, 0.1 g polyunsaturated fat, <0.1 g monounsaturated fat, 1 mg cholesterol, 9 g carbohydrate, 3 g protein, 30 mg sodium

EXCHANGES: ½ vegetable; ½ skim milk

French Onion Soup

◆

Here is a fast and easy version of onion soup that can be quite enjoyable. Swiss-type cheeses and provolone are usually melted on top of onion soup, but use whatever low-fat or fat-free cheese you prefer. If you have homemade beef stock, by all means use it, but the consommé also works well.

4 c. thinly sliced large yellow onions
2 tsp. sugar
2 cans (10½ oz. each) beef consommé with gelatin added
2 cans water
2 Tbsp. dry sherry
Optional: pinch of dry thyme
8 slices French bread
8 oz. low-fat or fat-free Swiss or Provolone cheese

Place onions and sugar in large saucepan with ¼ c. of the broth. Simmer for 5–10 minutes, or until onions begin to soften, stirring every minute or so. Add remaining ingredients except cheese and bread slices, and bring to a boil. Reduce heat, cover, and simmer 15–20 minutes longer, or until onions are very soft.

Preheat broiler.

To serve, line bottoms of ovenproof bowls with French bread slices. Distribute the broth and cooked onions evenly among the bowls. Top each serving with 1 oz. of the cheese, and place bowls under broiler until cheese starts to bubble and brown slightly. (If you don't have ovenproof bowls, place soup in regular bowls. Top with cheese and serve at once.)

YIELD: 8 servings

Each ¾ c. serving: 155 calories, 4.9 g fat (28.4% calories from fat), 2.6 g saturated fat, 0.2 g polyunsaturated fat, 0.4 g monounsaturated fat, 15 mg cholesterol, 16.1 g carbohydrate, 11.9 g protein, 679 mg sodium

EXCHANGES: 1 bread; 1½ lean meat

Quick and Easy Hot and Sour Soup

◆

Unlike many recipes for hot and sour soup, this soup can be made from ingredients that are available at any supermarket. And it's ready within thirty minutes. Use cremini mushrooms if they're available, and use cider vinegar if you don't have white vinegar on hand.

3 c. thinly sliced mushrooms
4 c. fat-free chicken stock or broth
1 Tbsp. low-sodium tamari or soy sauce
1 clove garlic, pressed

1 tsp. sugar

¼ tsp. white pepper

2 Tbsp. plus 1 tsp. white vinegar

3 oz. soft tofu cut into ¼-by-¾-inch slices

3 Tbsp. cornstarch mixed into ¼ c. cold water

2 egg whites, beaten with fork

1 tsp. sesame oil

In large saucepan, combine mushrooms, chicken stock, tamari or soy sauce, garlic, sugar, white pepper, and vinegar. Bring to a boil, reduce heat to low and simmer about 15 minutes, or until mushrooms are softened. Add tofu and cornstarch-water mixture, and stir until thickened. Slowly pour in egg whites in thin stream, stirring soup so that egg whites form ribbons. Add sesame oil and serve hot.

YIELD: 6 servings

Each 1 c. serving: 52 calories, 1.6 g fat (27% calories from fat), 0.2 g saturated fat, 0.8 g polyunsaturated fat, 0.5 g monounsaturated fat, 0 mg cholesterol, 6.7 g carbohydrate, 3.4 g protein, 186 mg sodium

EXCHANGES: 1½ vegetables; ½ fat

Creamy Mushroom Soup

◆

This easy homemade soup actually tastes better the second day. Make it ahead and refrigerate it, and reheat it before serving. Avoid boiling milk-based soups, as they can curdle or scorch if overheated.

Served topped with fat-free sour cream and fresh parsley, this soup is a tasty and attractive beginning to any meal. ■

2 lb. mushrooms, cleaned and thinly sliced
1 medium onion, chopped
2 Tbsp. fresh lemon juice
1½ tsp. salt (*omit* if using canned broth)
⅛ tsp. ground black pepper
3 c. fat-free chicken broth
3 c. skim milk
¼ c. plus 2 Tbsp. cornstarch
Optional garnish: 8 tsp. fat-free sour cream and 8 fresh
    parsley sprigs

In large saucepan, combine mushrooms, onion, lemon juice, salt, black pepper, and chicken broth. Bring to a boil, cover, and reduce heat to low. Simmer 20 minutes, or until mushrooms and onions are very soft.

Combine cornstarch and skim milk, and stir until no lumps remain. Pour mixture into soup, and heat until thickened. Remove from heat. If desired, top each serving with 1 tsp. fat-free sour cream and one parsley sprig.

YIELD: 8 servings

Each ¾ c. serving: 77 calories, 0.7 g fat (8.2% calories from fat), 0.2 g saturated fat, 0.2 g polyunsaturated fat, <0.1 g monounsaturated fat, 1 mg cholesterol, 13.6 g carbohydrate, 5.5 g protein, 450 mg sodium

EXCHANGES: ½ bread; ½ skim milk

"Wild" Mushroom Soup

———◆———

Although this recipe is similar to Creamy Mushroom Soup, it takes advantage of the newer varieties of mushrooms now on the market and is much heartier and richer than the creamy version. The Portobello and cremini mushrooms give this soup a beautiful dark brown broth.

It is fun to serve this soup in "bread bowls." To make the bowls, buy or bake one small round loaf for each serving; slice off the top and then scoop out the bread to form a ½-inch thick "bowl." Toast the bread bowls in a 350°F. oven for 15 minutes or until crusty, and then pour in the soup. If you'd like, use the top of the loaf as a lid for each bowl; then your guests will have a surprise waiting for them inside! After eating the soup, be sure to enjoy the bowl.

2 lb. mushrooms (Portobello, cremini, oyster, and/or
    shiitake), cleaned and thinly sliced
1 medium onion, chopped
2 Tbsp. fresh lemon juice
1½ t. salt (omit if using canned broth)
⅛ tsp. ground black pepper
3 c. fat-free chicken broth
¼ c. plus 2 Tbsp. cornstarch
3 c. water
Optional garnish: 8 tsp. fat-free sour cream and 8 fresh
    parsley sprigs

Combine mushrooms, onion, lemon juice, salt, and black pepper to chicken broth in saucepan. Bring to a boil, cover, and reduce heat to low. Simmer 20 minutes, or until mushrooms and onions are very soft.

Stir cornstarch into ½ c. of the water until no lumps

remain. Pour mixture into saucepan along with the
remaining 2½ c. water, and heat until soup becomes
thickened. Remove from heat and serve. If desired,
top each serving with 1 tsp. fat-free sour cream and a
parsley sprig.

YIELD: 8 servings

Each ¾ c. serving: 55 calories, 0.5 g fat (8.2% calories from
fat), <0.1 g saturated fat, 0.2 g polyunsaturated fat, <0.1 g
monounsaturated fat, 0 mg cholesterol, 11.6 g carbohydrate,
2.5 g protein, 403 mg sodium

EXCHANGES: 1 bread

Navy Bean Soup

———◆———

My mother made this soup every time it snowed, and it grew
to be one of my favorites. Now that research has shown that
the soluble fiber in beans reduces cholesterol levels, it's wise
to enjoy this soup often.

    1 pound dried navy beans
    8 c. water
    1 large onion, chopped, or 1 c. chopped scallions
    2 celery stalks, chopped
    2 carrots, chopped
    1½ c. potatoes, cut into ¼-inch to ½-inch cubes
    ¼ c. chopped lean ham (fat removed)
    3 chicken bouillon cubes
    2 bay leaves, crushed
    ⅛ tsp. ground black pepper

Pour beans into large pot. Add water until it is two to three times the depth of the beans. Heat, and let beans boil 2–3 minutes. Turn off heat, and let pot stand, covered, 30 minutes. Drain beans in colander, and pour them back into pot along with the 8 cups fresh water and the remaining ingredients. Bring to a rolling boil, and boil approximately 5 minutes. Reduce heat to low and cover. Simmer 1½ to 2 hours, or until beans are tender, stirring every 10–15 minutes.

If you prefer a thickened soup, pour off ½ to 1 c. soup, puree in food processor, and stir back into soup. The more of the mixture you puree, the thicker the soup will be. If it becomes too thick, add water until soup is of the right consistency. (Keeping pot covered during cooking will reduce evaporation.)

Y I E L D :   10 servings

Each ¾ c. serving: 208 calories, 1.2 g fat (5.2% calories from fat), 0.3 g saturated fat, 0.4 g polyunsaturated fat, 0.3 g monounsaturated fat, 3 mg cholesterol, 38 g carbohydrate, 13 g protein, 205 mg sodium

E X C H A N G E S :   1 extra-lean meat; 2 breads; 1 vegetable

Potato-Scallion Soup

◆

Potato soup is comforting and so easy to make, and most people always have the ingredients on hand. This version calls for scallions, but it's equally as good with onion or leeks.

For a down-home meal, I use scallions or onions and leave large chunks of potatoes in the soup. For a more elegant presentation I use leeks, and I puree the soup before serving it.

6 c. potatoes, peeled and cut into ½-in. cubes
1 c. chopped scallions, both green and white parts
⅓ c. finely chopped celery
3 Tbsp. diced lean ham
1–2 Tbsp. chopped fresh parsley
1 tsp. salt
2½ c. water
2½ c. skim milk
⅛ tsp. ground black pepper
Garnish: chopped green parts of scallions

Combine potatoes, scallions, celery, ham, parsley, salt, and water in large saucepan. Bring to a boil, cover, and reduce heat to medium. Boil slowly for about 10 minutes, or until potatoes are soft. Mash mixture with whisk to break apart some of the potatoes.

Add skim milk and black pepper to soup, and heat just to a boil. Remove from heat, and ladle into bowls. Garnish with chopped scallion tops.

YIELD: 8 servings

Each 6 oz. serving: 160 calories, 0.5 g fat (2.8% calories from

fat), 0.2 g saturated fat, 0.1 g polyunsaturated fat, 0.1 g
monounsaturated fat, 3 mg cholesterol, 33.5 g carbohydrate,
6.0 g protein, 364 mg sodium

EXCHANGES: 2 breads; 1 vegetable

Fresh Corn Soup

We enjoy this soup chilled. It's a little bit of trouble to make
but well worth the effort. I like it best with very little extra
flavoring, but it is good too with pimiento or chopped red
pepper.

    4 large ears corn
    2 qt. water
    1 tsp. salt
    ¼ tsp. ground black pepper
    ¼ tsp. dried tarragon leaves
    1 large onion, coarsely chopped
    2 cloves garlic
    Optional: 1 Tbsp. sugar (omit if corn is fresh and sweet)
    ½ c. skim milk powder
    Chopped parsley, fat-free sour cream, or roasted red
        pepper strips for garnish

Cut corn kernels from cobs and set kernels aside.
Place cobs in large pot with remaining ingredients
except corn kernels, skim milk powder, and garnish.
Bring to a boil, then reduce heat, and simmer 45
minutes. Remove cobs, and add corn kernels. Simmer
for another 15–20 minutes, or until kernels are tender.
Pour soup mixture into blender or food processor,

a bit at a time, and process until smooth. Strain the mixture, whisk in skim milk powder, and adjust seasonings to taste. Refrigerate until ready to serve. Top with chopped parsley, dollop of fat-free sour cream, or roasted red pepper strips.

YIELD: 6 servings

Each 1 c. serving: 89 calories, 0.8 g fat (8.1% calories from fat), 0.2 g saturated fat, 0.4 g polyunsaturated fat, 0.2 g monounsaturated fat, 1 mg cholesterol, 18.9 g carbohydrate, 4.2 g protein, 396 mg sodium

EXCHANGES: 1 bread; 1 vegetable

Honeydew Melon Soup

———◆———

A simple but delicious summer soup. If you like, try it with cantaloupe instead of honeydew, but either way, be sure to use fully ripened melons for this soup.

    8 c. ripe honeydew chunks
    4–6 fresh mint leaves
    Optional: 1–2 Tbsp. honey or sugar
    1 c. plain nonfat yogurt
    Mint sprigs for garnish

Place honeydew and mint in bowl of food processor, and process until smooth. Taste and add the honey or sugar, if needed. Refrigerate until chilled. Just before serving, whisk in yogurt. Garnish each serving with sprig of mint.

YIELD: 5 cups (approx. 6 servings)

Each serving: 101 calories, 0.3 g fat (2.7% calories from fat), <0.1 g saturated fat, <0.1 g monounsaturated fat, <0.1 g polyunsaturated fat, 0 mg cholesterol, 23.4 g carbohydrate, 3.2 g protein, 51 mg sodium

EXCHANGES: 1 fruit; ½ skim milk

MAIN DISHES

◆

The main dish is the highlight of the meal—the element around which we plan the rest of the meal.

Here is a large array of main dishes—from poultry, seafood, and lean beef and pork to sandwiches and meatless dishes. Some recipes are for traditional American foods while others feature foods from different ethnic cuisines.

No matter what the occasion—a simple and quick dinner for the family or an elegant dinner party for special guests—you should find something here that is perfect for your occasion.

POULTRY

Marinated Turkey Breast
with Orange Glaze

———◆———

When I was growing up, turkey was served only on Thanksgiving and Christmas. It was served with oysters and ham, but it remained the highlight of the meal. In this recipe, I marinate the breast to help preserve its natural juices, and I cook it only until it is no longer pink near the bone. An orange glaze adds a finishing touch.

1 turkey breast (6 pounds)

Marinade:
1 c. plain nonfat yogurt
1 small onion, coarsely chopped
½–1 tsp. salt
1 tsp. poultry seasoning
½ t. dried rosemary

Glaze:
1 Tbsp. cornstarch
½ c. water
½ c. frozen orange juice concentrate, thawed
½ c. dark corn syrup
½ lb. white seedless grapes
½ lb. red seedless grapes
Optional: 4–6 fresh orange slices, seeds removed

Remove skin and all visible fat from the turkey breast and set it aside.

To prepare marinade: place yogurt, onion, salt, and poultry seasoning in bowl of food processor or blender, and process until smooth. Stir in rosemary. Place turkey breast in covered bowl or waterproof plastic bag. Pour marinade over turkey, covering entire surface. Marinate in refrigerator at least 4 hours.

Preheat oven to 350°F. Remove turkey from refrigerator and place in baking pan, discarding extra marinade. Bake turkey about 20 minutes per pound (2 hours for 6 lb. breast), or until meat is no longer pink near bone. (Overcooking will toughen meat and cause it to dry out.) Remove turkey from oven.

Near end of cooking time, prepare glaze: In small saucepan, stir cornstarch into water until smooth, and add orange juice concentrate and corn syrup. Cook mixture on high, stirring constantly, until sauce begins to boil and thicken. Immediately remove from heat, continuing to stir until sauce stops bubbling. Stir in white and red grapes, coating them well with the glaze.

Place turkey on platter. Remove grapes from glaze with slotted spoon and arrange around turkey. Pour sauce over turkey breast. Place orange slices on top as garnish, if desired.

YIELD: 20 servings

Each 3 oz. serving: 172 calories, 1.5 g fat (7.8% calories from fat), 0.3 g saturated fat, 0.2 g polyunsaturated fat, 0.2 g monounsaturated fat, 75 mg cholesterol, 13.0 g carbohydrate, 27.6 g protein, 83 mg sodium

EXCHANGES: 3½ extra-lean meats; 1 fruit

Crispy Oven-"Fried" Chicken

———◆———

This recipe is a favorite with my children and their friends. Make it as spicy as you wish by adding extra seasoned salt and black pepper.

1½ c. bread crumbs
½ tsp. seasoned salt, or more to taste
Ground black pepper to taste
9 chicken pieces, skinned and trimmed of all fat

Preheat oven to 350°F., and lightly coat large baking pan with vegetable oil spray.

Mix bread crumbs with seasoned salt and pepper. Taste crumb mixture and add more seasoning if desired. Pat crumbs onto top of chicken pieces, and place chicken in baking pan.

Bake 30 minutes. Increase oven temperature to 400°F., and cook chicken another 20–30 minutes, or until meat is no longer pink near bone on largest pieces.

YIELD: 9 servings

Each serving: 100 calories, 2.3 g fat (20.7% calories from fat), 0.6 g saturated fat, 0.5 g polyunsaturated fat, 0.6 g monounsaturated fat, 46 mg cholesterol, 3.8 g carbohydrate, 14.9 g protein, 156 mg sodium

EXCHANGES: 2 extra-lean meats; ⅓ bread

Spicy Turkey Chili

◆

This chili's spicy aroma will fill your house and linger through-out the evening. Serve it as a main dish with hot bread, fruit, and salad for a simple, satisfying meal, or offer it as an accompaniment to other favorite foods. You can make this chili with chicken instead of turkey if you like.

1½ lb. turkey breast, cut into ¼-inch cubes, or 1½ lb.
    ground turkey (93 + % lean)
1 medium green bell pepper, seeded and chopped
1 large onion, chopped
1 can (28 oz.) crushed tomatoes
2 cloves garlic, pressed
2 bay leaves, crumbled
3 Tbsp. chili powder
1 Tbsp. ground cumin
¼ tsp. ground black pepper
2 cans (16 oz. each) kidney beans, with liquid
Salt to taste

Lightly coat 8-quart pan with vegetable oil spray. Brown turkey with green pepper and onion. Remove turkey from pan and pour off juices. Replace turkey in pan, add remaining ingredients, and bring to a boil. Lower heat, stir well, and simmer, covered, 15 min-utes, stirring every few minutes to prevent sticking. If desired, add salt to taste.

YIELD: 10 servings

Each ¾ c. serving: 191 calories, 2.1 g fat (9.5% calories from fat), 0.4 g saturated fat, 0.6 g polyunsaturated fat, 0.3 g

monounsaturated fat, 41 mg cholesterol, 22 g carbohydrate, 23 g protein, 559 mg sodium

EXCHANGES: 2½ extra-lean meat; 1½ bread

VARIATION: For Meatless Chili, follow instructions above, but omit turkey and salt and use four cans kidney beans instead of two. Drain three of the cans of beans, and use the last can undrained. If desired, substitute garbanzo or black beans for some of the kidney beans.

YIELD FOR MEATLESS CHILI: 10 servings

Each ¾ c. serving: 160 calories, 1.2 g total fat (6.3% calories from fat), 0.1 g saturated fat, 0.4 g polyunsaturated fat, <0.1 g monounsaturated fat, 0 mg cholesterol, 30 g carbohydrate, 9 g protein, 685 mg sodium

EXCHANGES: 2 breads; ½ lean meat

Turkey-Vegetable Loaf

◆

This recipe calls for spinach or zucchini, but feel free to try other vegetables and combinations of vegetables, too.

1¼ lb. ground turkey (93 + % lean)
1 small onion, grated
1 c. fresh spinach or grated zucchini, well packed
1 large tomato, chopped
¼ c. minced celery
2 cloves garlic, pressed
½ tsp. salt
1 Tbsp. Worcestershire sauce
¼ tsp. ground black pepper
4 slices fresh bread ground into crumbs (about 2 c.)
2 egg whites
½ c. ketchup

Preheat oven to 350°F. Combine all ingredients except ketchup, and mix well. Press into 9½-by-5½-inch loaf pan and spread ketchup over top. Bake 1 hour, or until turkey loaf is no longer pink in middle. Remove from oven, drain off juices, and let sit 5–10 minutes before serving.

YIELD: 10 servings

Each slice: 118 calories, 2.2 g fat (15.2% calories from fat), 0.7 g saturated fat, 0.7 g polyunsaturated fat, 0.6 g mono-unsaturated fat, 36 mg cholesterol, 9.5 g carbohydrate, 15.1 g protein, 326 mg sodium

EXCHANGES: 1½ extra-lean meats; 2 vegetables

Chicken Cacciatore

—————◆—————

Chicken Cacciatore means "Hunter's Chicken" in Italian. It's an easy recipe that tastes wonderful with pasta, a simple salad, and fresh bread. For a really fast meal, use turkey cutlets; because they are thinner, they cook faster.

4 boneless chicken breasts (or turkey cutlets) (about
   1 lb.)
4 cloves garlic, pressed
1½ c. crushed tomatoes
½ c. dry red wine
Optional: ½ tsp. salt
½ tsp. dried basil leaves, crushed
¼ tsp. dried sweet marjoram
6 mushrooms, thinly sliced

Lightly coat nonstick skillet with vegetable oil spray. Brown chicken breasts on both sides. Lower heat and sauté until thickest part of breast is no longer pink inside. Transfer chicken to serving plate.

Add remaining ingredients to skillet and heat, stirring, until bubbly and slightly thickened. Return chicken to skillet and spoon sauce over it. Reduce heat, and cook, covered, until chicken and sauce are both hot.

YIELD: 4 servings

Each serving: 178 calories, 1.6 g fat (8.1% calories from fat), 0.4 g saturated fat, 0.4 g polyunsaturated fat, 0.4 g monounsaturated fat, 66 mg cholesterol, 8.2 g carbohydrate, 27.5 g protein, 291 mg sodium

EXCHANGES: 3 extra-lean meats; 1½ vegetables

Chicken Marsala

If you don't have sweet Marsala wine, consider buying an inexpensive bottle for this recipe. Serve Chicken Marsala with hot pasta—linguine and penne are our favorites—fruit, salad, and French or Italian bread, and you'll have a delightful Italian meal.

This dish is also good when it's made with turkey cutlets.

4 boneless chicken breasts (about 1 lb.)
1 c. sliced mushrooms
2 cloves garlic, pressed
¾ c. sweet Marsala wine
1 Tbsp. finely chopped fresh parsley, or 1 tsp. dried
Optional: Salt and ground black pepper to taste
Optional: 1 Tbsp. cornstarch mixed with 1 Tbsp. water

Lightly coat skillet with vegetable oil spray. Brown chicken on both sides. Reduce heat, cover, and sauté until no pink remains in middle of breasts. Transfer chicken to plate, add mushrooms and garlic to skillet, and sauté until tender. Add Marsala and parsley, and simmer, uncovered, until liquid is reduced by half. Taste and add salt and pepper if desired. If you wish a thicker sauce, stir in cornstarch-water mixture slowly just until you reach the desired thickness. You probably won't need all of it. Serve chicken hot with sauce.

YIELD: 4 servings

Each serving: 151 calories, 1.3 g fat (7.7% calories from fat), 0.3 g saturated fat, 0.3 g polyunsaturated fat, 0.3 g

monounsaturated fat, 57 mg cholesterol, 3.2 g carbohydrate, 23.2 g protein, 70 mg sodium

EXCHANGES: 3 extra-lean meats; ½ vegetable

Tandoori Chicken

———◆———

This recipe is one of my all-time favorites. Inspired by the recipe in Madhur Jaffrey's *Invitation to Indian Cooking*, I came up with this fat-free marinade and simplified the dish for a quicker meal. The original contained twenty-three ingredients—but, oh, it was so good! Serve this dish hot with rice or Indian potatoes.

1 medium onion, quartered
1 c. plain nonfat yogurt
2 Tbsp. lemon juice
2 cloves garlic
1 tsp. ground cumin
1 Tbsp. ground coriander
1 tsp. ground turmeric
1–2 tsp. salt
¼ tsp. ground black pepper
¼ tsp. ground cinnamon
Optional: ½ tsp. cayenne
6 chicken breasts

Place all ingredients except chicken in bowl of food processor or blender and process until smooth. Pour mixture over chicken pieces in large bowl or large sealable plastic bag. Refrigerate at least two hours (four or more is better), stirring (or shaking bag) at least once during the marinating period.

Remove chicken, reserving marinade and place on preheated grill on low to medium heat. Cook until chicken is no longer pink near bone (20–25 minutes), turning frequently to prevent burning. If desired, redip chicken pieces in marinade during cooking for extra moisture and flavor. (This can also be cooked in a 350°F. oven for 45 minutes to 1 hour.)

YIELD: 6 servings

Each serving: 122 calories, 1.2 g fat (8.9% calories from fat), 0.3 g saturated fat, 0.3 g polyunsaturated fat, 0.3 g monounsaturated fat, 50 mg cholesterol, 4.6 g carbohydrate, 22.1 g protein, 399 mg sodium

EXCHANGES: 2½ extra-lean meats; ½ skim milk

Chicken-Yogurt Curry

Here's a wonderful recipe given to me by my good friend Julia Taylor of Burke, Virginia. This is an ideal dish for a crowd, since it can be doubled or tripled and you can make it ahead of time. Serve over any long-grain rice (basmati is Julia's favorite) with a salad or vegetable, bread, and dessert.

If you bone your chicken before cooking, it will cook much faster.

1½ lb. chicken pieces
1 medium onion, quartered
3 cloves garlic
1 tsp. minced fresh ginger
½ c. cilantro leaves
1 tsp. ground turmeric

½ tsp. chili powder

¼ tsp. ground black pepper

¼ tsp. ground cinnamon

¼ tsp. salt

½ c. plain nonfat yogurt

2 fresh or canned tomatoes, diced

Clean chicken, remove skin, and set chicken aside. Place onion, garlic, ginger, and cilantro in bowl of blender or food processor, and puree. Lightly coat nonstick pan with vegetable oil spray. Transfer onion mixture to pan, and cook about 5 minutes over medium heat. Add spices and salt, and cook 1 minute longer. Mix in yogurt and tomatoes, and cook another 2–3 minutes.

Add chicken to pan, and cook, covered, until chicken becomes tender and is no longer pink near the bone.

YIELD: 6 servings

Each serving: 117 calories, 2.4 g fat (18.5% calories from fat), 0.6 g saturated fat, 0.6 g polyunsaturated fat, 0.7 g monounsaturated fat, 53 mg cholesterol, 4.7 g carbohydrate, 18.6 g protein, 162 mg sodium

EXCHANGES: 2½ extra-lean meats; 1 vegetable

Oriental Chicken Salad

◆

For potluck dinners I often double this recipe and arrange the salad attractively on a large platter. It always receives rave reviews.

4 boneless chicken breasts
1 Tbsp. low-sodium soy or tamari sauce
2 cloves garlic, pressed
1 head romaine, cleaned, dried, and cut into ¾-inch
   slices
3 scallions, thinly sliced
½ lb. fresh bean sprouts
1 large red bell pepper, seeded and cut into thin strips
1 Tbsp. toasted sesame seeds

Dressing:
1 Tbsp. low-sodium soy or tamari sauce
2 tsp. sesame oil
1 clove garlic, pressed
1 tsp. minced fresh ginger

Place chicken breasts in baking dish. Combine soy sauce with pressed garlic cloves and spread mixture over all surfaces of chicken. Cover dish and refrigerate at least 2 hours.

Grill or bake chicken just until no pink remains. Thinly slice each breast against the grain.

Place romaine in one bowl. Reserve ¼ c. of the scallions for garnish, and combine remaining scallions with the bean sprouts in second bowl.

Mix together all the dressing ingredients. Divide the dressing between the two bowls, and toss the ingredients in each bowl separately.

Make a bed of romaine on each of four plates. Top with bean sprout–scallion mixture. Arrange chicken strips on top. Sprinkle with the ¼ c. reserved scallions, and lay the red pepper strips attractively over the top. Sprinkle toasted sesame seeds over all.

YIELD: 4 servings

Each serving: 259 calories, 8.2 g fat (28.4% calories from fat), 1.7 g saturated fat, 2.6 g polyunsaturated fat, 2.9 g monounsaturated fat, 96 mg cholesterol, 7.5 g carbohydrate, 38.3 g protein, 467 mg sodium

EXCHANGES: 4 lean meat; 1 vegetable

Chicken Biryani

———◆———

This was the first Indian dish I ever tasted, and it quickly became one of my all-time favorites. For the best flavor, use basmati rice.

    2 large onions, coarsely chopped
    4 cloves garlic, peeled
    1 cube (1 inch by 1 inch) fresh ginger, peeled and
        coarsely chopped
    1 tsp. ground coriander
    1 tsp. ground cumin
    ½ tsp. turmeric
    ¼ tsp. ground black pepper
    1 tsp. salt
    2 Tbsp. fresh lemon juice
    1 c. fat-free plain yogurt

2 lb. boneless, skinless chicken breast, cut into strips ¼
    inch to ½ inch wide
½ c. raisins
4 c. hot cooked rice
Parsley sprigs, grapes, and orange or lemon wedges

Place onions, garlic, spices, salt, and lemon juice in
bowl of food processor or blender. Process until
smooth, stir into yogurt, and add chicken strips. Refrigerate mixture at least 2 hours.

Lightly coat large skillet with vegetable oil spray,
add chicken and yogurt mixtures, and bring to a boil.
Reduce heat to low, add raisins, and simmer, stirring
occasionally, 20 minutes or until meat is no longer
pink in center.

Place hot cooked rice in middle of platter, and top
with hot chicken and sauce, or, if desired, combine
rice with chicken mixture before serving. Top with
parsley sprigs and garnish rim of platter with grapes
and orange or lemon wedges.

YIELD: 8 servings

Each serving: 296 calories, 1.7 g fat (5.2% calories from
fat), 0.4 g saturated fat, 0.4 g polyunsaturated fat, 0.4 g
monounsaturated fat, 66 mg cholesterol, 38.3 g carbohydrate,
30.7 g protein, 364 mg sodium

EXCHANGES: 3½ extra-lean meat; 2 breads; ½ fruit

Turkey Fajitas

———◆———

This is one of my favorite "hectic day" recipes. When shopping for tortillas, be sure to check the fat content, as I've seen it vary from zero to four grams of fat per tortilla. You can make these fajitas with chicken cutlets instead of turkey for a tasty change of pace.

- 1 lb. turkey breast cutlets, cut into strips ¼ to
  ½ inch wide
- 1 large green bell pepper, cut into strips
- 1 large red bell pepper, cut into strips
- 1 medium onion, cut into thin wedges
- ½ tsp. salt
- ¼ tsp. ground black pepper
- Optional: ⅛ tsp. ground red pepper or cayenne
- 12 flour tortillas, 7 to 8 inches in diameter
- Picante sauce

Lightly coat a nonstick pan with vegetable oil spray. Sauté turkey breast strips until all pink has disappeared. Add peppers and onion, and sauté until onion is tender. Stir in salt, black pepper, and, if you wish, red pepper.

Wrap stack of tortillas with paper towels, and microwave until hot. Place top tortilla on work surface and spread turkey mixture down middle of tortilla. Top with picante sauce, and roll into fajita. Repeat with remaining tortillas.

YIELD: 12 fajitas

Each fajita: 162 calories, 2.8 g fat (15.6% calories from fat), 0.5 g saturated fat, 1.1 g polyunsaturated fat, 1.1 g

monounsaturated fat, 25 mg cholesterol, 21.3 g carbohydrate, 12.3 g protein, 312 mg sodium

EXCHANGES: 1 lean meat; 1 bread; 1 vegetable

Turkey Sausage

———◆———

Judy Wolff of Ann Arbor, Michigan, uses this sausage in chili, spaghetti, tacos, pizza, casseroles, and anywhere she used to use ground beef.

Feel free to vary the spices in your sausage. Add ¼ tsp. ground cumin, ¼ tsp. dried oregano, and 1 or 2 pinches crushed red pepper to make a Mexican sausage. Make Italian sausage by adding ½ tsp. fennel seed. I like to add extra garlic and 1 tsp. mustard seeds for a kielbasa-type sausage.

When you choose ground turkey, be sure to read the label; ground turkey can contain as much as five or six grams of fat per ounce or as little as one or two grams, depending on the brand.

    1 lb. ground turkey (93 + % lean)
    2 cloves garlic, minced
    ½ onion, finely chopped
    2 Tbsp. oat bran
    ½ tsp. salt

Mix together all ingredients and refrigerate several hours or overnight to develop flavor. Leave sausage in bulk or shape into patties. Use within two days or freeze for later use.

YIELD: 16 servings

Each 1 oz. serving: 40 calories, 1.0 g fat (22.5% calories from fat), 0.2 g saturated fat, 0.2 g polyunsaturated fat, 0.1 g monounsaturated fat, 25 mg cholesterol, 0.5 g carbohydrate, 6.8 g protein, 85 mg sodium

EXCHANGES: 1 lean meat

Country Breakfast Sausage

◆

When I was young, my family raised hogs, and we all looked forward to hog-killing day and the fresh sausage my mother would make. The seasoning in this sausage is similar to the blend that my mother used.

1 lb. ground turkey (93 + % lean)
2 cloves garlic, minced
½ tsp. salt
½ tsp. ground black pepper
Optional: ⅛ tsp. ground red pepper
1 tsp. crushed sage
2 Tbsp. oat bran

Combine all ingredients and shape mixture into patties. Refrigerate for use within two days, or freeze for later use.

YIELD: 16 servings

Each 1 oz. serving: 40 calories, 1.0 g fat (22.5% calories from fat), 0.2 g saturated fat, 0.2 g polyunsaturated fat, 0.1 g monounsaturated fat, 25 mg cholesterol, 0.5 g carbohydrate, 6.8 g protein, 85 mg sodium

EXCHANGES: 1 extra-lean meat

Curried Grilled Chicken Salad

———◆———

Chicken salad has always been one of my favorite foods, but I rarely make it because of the time involved in cooking and boning the chicken and because of all of the fat in the mayonnaise. This low-fat salad is much faster. It's also ideal for entertaining, for a potluck get-together, or for just you and your family!

  1 lb. chicken breast, boned, skinned, and cut into strips
  ½ plain nonfat yogurt
  1 tsp. curry powder
  ¼ tsp. salt
  ¼ tsp. cumin seeds
  1 tsp. sesame seeds
  20–30 frozen green peas
  ½ medium-sized fresh tomato, cut into ½-inch chunks

Cook chicken strips on aluminum foil over grill, or sauté them indoors in nonstick skillet, just until the meat is no longer pink inside. Set aside to cool.

Place cooked chicken in mixing bowl with yogurt, seasonings, and peas, and combine well. Just before serving, toss in tomato chunks.

YIELD: 6 servings

Each serving: 154 calories, 3.1 g fat (18.1% calories from fat), 0.8 g saturated fat, 0.7 g polyunsaturated fat, 1.1 g monounsaturated fat, 64 mg cholesterol, 4.6 g carbohydrate, 25.6 g protein, 172 mg sodium

EXCHANGES: 3 extra-lean meat; 1 vegetable

SEAFOOD

Poached Salmon Squares

◆

Anyone who makes these salmon squares once will probably make them again and again. This is a great "make-ahead" entrée. Assemble and wrap the squares early in the day, and cook them just before serving. Buy only the freshest salmon available.

    3 lb. red salmon fillets
    ½ lb. fresh spinach leaves, washed well
    2 jars (6 oz. each) whole pimientos
    Salt and pepper to taste

Remove skin and any remaining bones from salmon fillets. Slice through fillets lengthwise, so that each fillet becomes two thinner fillets. Cut fish into 16 squares. Make 8 sets of squares, matching the 2 squares in each set (as closely as possible) in size and shape.

Remove top layer of the first set. Place three or four spinach leaves on the fish, followed by a layer of pimiento, cutting the spinach and pimiento to fit the shape of the salmon. Place top layer back on salmon to form a sandwich.

Repeat for each double salmon square. When all are completed, sprinkle salt and pepper over them and wrap each double square tightly in aluminum foil. Place wrapped fish squares in a large pan of simmering water. Cook 10 minutes, or until fish flakes with fork.

YIELD: 8 servings

Each serving: 182 calories, 5.2 g fat (25.9% calories from fat), 0.9 g saturated fat, 2.1 g polyunsaturated fat, 1.4 g monounsaturated fat, 76 mg cholesterol, 2.4 g carbohydrate, 30.0 g protein, 121 mg sodium

EXCHANGES: 4 extra-lean meats; ½ vegetable

Stuffed Fish Rolls

------◆------

1 pound orange roughy or flounder fillets
1½ c. fine bread crumbs
½ tsp. dried sage leaves, crushed
⅛ tsp. ground black pepper
2 Tbsp. finely chopped onion
1 Tbsp. minced fresh parsley, or 1 tsp. parsley flakes
1 tomato, thinly sliced
3 Tbsp. lemon juice
Optional: Salt and pepper
Optional: White wine (approx. ½ c.)
4 fresh parsley sprigs
4 lemon wedges
½ tsp. honey

Preheat oven to 350°F., and lightly coat baking dish with vegetable oil spray.

Cut fish into four portions, and lay portions flat. Combine bread crumbs, sage, black pepper, chopped onion, and parsley. Top each fish portion with crumb mixture, dividing mixture evenly among portions. Roll fish up from end to end and tie each roll closed with 1 or 2 pieces of string.

Place fish rolls in pan and top with tomato slices and lemon juice. If desired, sprinkle fish rolls lightly with salt and black pepper. Pour wine into pan to ¼-inch depth, if desired. Bake 15 minutes, or until fish begins to flake throughout.

Remove pan from oven, cut strings, and garnish each portion with parsley sprig and lemon wedge. If any juices remain in bottom of pan, pour them into small bowl and stir in the honey; serve as sauce over fish portions.

Y I E L D : 4 servings

Each serving: 184 calories, 2.0 g fat (9.8% calories from fat), 0.5 g saturated fat, 0.4 g polyunsaturated fat, 0.3 g monounsaturated fat, 55 mg cholesterol, 13 g carbohydrate, 23.5 g protein, 186 mg sodium

E X C H A N G E S : 3 extra-lean meats; 1 bread

Marinated Seafood Kebabs

◆

This is a quick, attractive main dish that only looks like a lot of work. For an easy after-work meal, put the ingredients in the marinade in the morning, and arrange them on skewers in the afternoon while you're preheating the grill. If you use wooden skewers, remember to soak them for at least 30 minutes before using them.

1 pound monkfish, tuna, swordfish, or other firm-fleshed
    fish, cut into 1-inch chunks
6 jumbo shrimp, peeled except for tail and deveined
1 large green bell pepper, cut into 1-inch chunks

2 large, firm tomatoes cut into 1-inch chunks, or
   12 cherry tomatoes
1 large onion, peeled and cut into 1-inch chunks
6 oz. bottled fat-free Italian dressing
12 large fresh mushrooms
Hot cooked rice

Place fish, shrimp, green pepper, tomato, and onion in large bowl or sealable plastic bag. Pour Italian dressing over all, distributing it well. Refrigerate, covered or sealed, at least 4 hours. Stir mixture once during marinating period.

Preheat grill. Remove fish, shrimp, and vegetables from marinade, and thread onto 6 skewers along with mushrooms, alternating colors. Grill on medium heat for 10–15 minutes, turning every few minutes, until fish is cooked through.

Serve hot over rice.

YIELD: **6 servings**

Each serving: 105 calories, 1.9 g fat (16.3% calories from fat), <0.1 g saturated fat, 0.2 g polyunsaturated fat, <0.1 g monounsaturated fat, 38 mg cholesterol, 5.1 g carbohydrate, 17.0 g protein, 126 mg sodium

EXCHANGES: **2 extra-lean meats; 1 vegetable**

Sesame "Fried" Fish Squares

──────◆──────

If you miss having a "fried fish night" at your house, try this recipe with your favorite variety of fish—orange roughy and cod are both good. Take care not to overcook these squares or the fish will become tough.

    1 lb. fish fillets
    ½ c. whole wheat bread crumbs
    1 Tbsp. sesame seeds
    1 egg white mixed with 1 Tbsp. water
    4 lemon wedges
    4 fresh parsley sprigs
    Optional: fat-free tartar sauce

Preheat oven to 400°F., and lightly coat large baking sheet with vegetable oil spray.

Cut fish fillets into portion-sized squares and set aside. Combine bread crumbs and sesame seeds in small bowl. Dip fish portions in egg white mixture, and coat with bread crumb mixture. Place fish on prepared baking sheet, making sure portions do not touch one another. Bake 10–12 minutes, depending upon thickness, until fish flakes throughout.

Top each serving with lemon wedge and parsley sprig. Serve with fat-free tartar sauce, if desired.

YIELD: 4 servings

Each serving: 164 calories, 2.8 g fat (15.4% calories from fat), 0.4 g saturated fat, 0.7 g polyunsaturated fat, 1.4 g monounsaturated fat, 28 mg cholesterol, 10.4 g carbohydrate, 23 g protein, 215 mg sodium

EXCHANGES: 3 extra-lean meats; ½ bread

Sea Leg Imperial

◆

Each serving of the original version of this recipe contained 46 grams of fat. This version, with only 4.3 grams of fat per serving, is almost as good. It's a splendid make-ahead dish. I· frequently take it to potluck dinners, and people always ask for the recipe. Serve hot with a salad and French or Italian bread. You can use imitation crab or lobster flakes instead of Sea Legs, if you wish.

   2 c. skim milk
   ¼ c. all-purpose flour
   1–2 Tbsp. dry sherry or dry white wine
   ½ tsp. salt
   1 tsp. Worcestershire sauce
   2 tsp. dry mustard
   ½ tsp. parsley flakes
   ¾ c. plain nonfat yogurt
   1 lb. Sea Legs
   3 c. hot cooked rice or pasta

Combine milk and flour in heavy saucepan, whisking or stirring until flour is well dispersed. Add sherry, salt, Worcestershire sauce, and mustard, and heat, stirring constantly, until sauce thickens and just begins to bubble. Remove from heat, and stir in parsley, yogurt, and Sea Legs. Serve hot over rice or pasta.

VARIATION: To make Imperial Casserole, place sea-food-yogurt mixture in casserole dish, and top with ½ c. bread crumbs. Refrigerate until ready to bake. Place casserole in 350°F. oven 30 minutes before serving, and heat until bubbly around edges and hot in the middle. Serve over rice or noodles.

YIELD: 4 servings

Each ½ c. serving with ½ c. rice: 380 calories, 4.3 g fat (10.2% calories from fat), 2.0 g saturated fat, 0.6 g polyunsaturated fat, 0.3 g monounsaturated fat, 122 mg cholesterol, 40 g carbohydrate, 41 g protein, 720 mg sodium

EXCHANGES: 4 extra-lean meats; 2 breads; 1 skim milk

BEEF AND PORK

Hearty Beef Stew

◆

This stew makes a hearty, nurturing meal for a blustery night. Served with piping hot bread and a crisp green salad, this is one of my family's favorite cold-weather meals. This stew can be made ahead and frozen.

2 lb. lean stew beef, cut into 1-inch cubes, all fat removed
2 c. water, or 1½ c. water plus ½ c. dry red wine
4 large potatoes, peeled and cut into ¾-inch cubes
2 medium celery stalks, chopped
2 large carrots, peeled and cut into ¼-inch slices
2 small onions, peeled and coarsely chopped
1 large tomato, cored and cut into ½-inch chunks
½ Tbsp. Worcestershire sauce
2 bay leaves, crumbled

2 beef bouillon cubes
½ tsp. salt
½ tsp. ground black pepper
6 Tbsp. all-purpose flour
½ c. water
1 c. frozen peas

Place beef cubes and water, or water and wine, in Dutch oven or large pot. Bring to a boil, reduce heat to medium, cover, and cook about 10 minutes, or until meat is cooked through. Drain beef, reserving liquid. Defat juices by cooling liquid and then skimming solid fat from surface, or by using a gravy skimmer.

Return beef and juices to Dutch oven. Add potatoes, celery, carrots, onions, tomato, Worcestershire sauce, bay leaves, bouillon cubes, salt, and pepper. Bring to a boil, stir, reduce heat, and simmer, *covered*, for approximately 1 hour, stirring every 10 minutes or so to prevent sticking.

When all vegetables are tender, drain stew in colander, catching juices in 2–4 qt. saucepan. Place saucepan over high heat. Mix the 6 Tbsp. flour into the ½ c. water, stirring to form a very smooth paste. Add paste to saucepan slowly, stirring with spoon or whisk until broth begins to boil and sauce coats spoon well. You may not need all of the paste.

Remove pan from heat. Return stew to Dutch oven, pour sauce back into stew mixture, and add frozen peas. Taste for seasoning and add more salt or pepper if desired. Heat through and serve at once, or store in refrigerator up to 3 days.

Y I E L D : 12 servings

Each ¾ c. serving: 201 calories, 3.5 g fat (15.7% calories from fat), 1.2 g saturated fat, 0.2 g polyunsaturated fat, 1.4 g monounsaturated fat, 40 mg cholesterol, 23 g carbohydrate, 19 g protein, 156 mg sodium

E X C H A N G E S : 2 extra-lean meats; 2 vegetables; 1 bread

Beef and Broccoli with Peanut Sauce

◆

This colorful dish features the flavors of Indonesia—soy sauce, peanuts, garlic, and molasses. Make it spicy, if you wish, by adding ground red pepper, or cayenne. Or make it meatless by omitting the beef and adding 2 cups of fresh cauliflower florets.

1½ c. uncooked white rice
3 c. boiling water
4 cloves garlic, pressed or minced
2 Tbsp. molasses
2 Tbsp. soy sauce
2 Tbsp. creamy peanut butter
Optional: ⅛ tsp. ground red pepper
Juice of ½ lemon
⅓ c. water
1 lb. very lean boneless beef sirloin, cut into slices
    ¼ inch thick
2 c. broccoli florets
1 red bell pepper, cut into strips
1 Tbsp. cornstarch mixed with 1 Tbsp. water

Add rice to boiling water, and cook while preparing rest of meal.

In small bowl, combine garlic, molasses, soy sauce, peanut butter, ground red pepper if desired, lemon juice, and the ⅓ c. water.

Lightly coat nonstick skillet with vegetable oil spray. Sauté beef until no pink remains. Add broccoli, sweet red pepper strips, and peanut butter mixture, stirring well. When broccoli is bright green and tender, add just enough cornstarch-water mixture to thicken sauce slightly. Serve hot over the cooked rice.

YIELD: 6 servings

Each serving: 274 calories, 6.3 g fat (20.7% calories from fat), 1.8 g saturated fat, 1.0 g polyunsaturated fat, 2.7 g monounsaturated fat, 40 mg cholesterol, 35.0 g carbohydrate, 19.2 g protein, 410 mg sodium

EXCHANGES: 2 lean meats; 1 bread; 1 vegetable; 1 fruit

"Fried" Potatoes and Ham

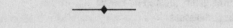

These potatoes remind me of the ones my mother served when I was a child. Serve them with a fruit and a green vegetable for dinner, or enjoy them with fruit and toast for breakfast.

    1 pkg. (24 oz.) frozen Ore Ida Potatoes O'Brien (with
        onions and peppers), thawed
    1 pkg. (6 oz.) lean breakfast ham (1 g fat per oz.), diced
    ¼ c. plus 1 c. water
    Optional: ¼ tsp. salt
    Optional: ⅛ tsp. ground black pepper

Lightly coat skillet with vegetable oil spray. Add potatoes and ham to skillet along with the ¼ c. water. Taste and add salt and pepper if desired. When water has evaporated, add the remaining 1 c. water, stir, and cover. Reduce heat, and simmer about 5 minutes, until all water has been absorbed and potatoes have begun to brown slightly. Serve hot.

YIELD: 6 servings

Each serving: 137 calories, 3.3 g fat (21.7% calories from fat), 7 mg cholesterol, 18.2 g carbohydrate, 9.3 g protein, 437 mg sodium

EXCHANGES: 1 lean meat; 1 bread

VARIATION: For a meatless version, omit the ham. If you like, substitute 2 Tbsp. soybean-based imitation bacon bits or ¼ to ½ tsp. liquid smoke.

Ham Steak with Cranberry Sauce

———◆———

Cranberry sauce turns this ham dish into real company fare that you can prepare in 30 minutes. For a lovely presentation, serve the ham steaks on a large platter surrounded with roasted potato wedges. When fresh or frozen cranberries aren't available, substitute dried cranberries soaked in water for 30 minutes before measuring.

    2½ lb. lean boneless lower-salt cooked ham steaks,
        trimmed of all visible fat
    2 c. apple cider or juice
    ½ c. bourbon
    ¼ c. balsamic vinegar
    ¼ c. finely chopped onion
    1 c. plus ½ c. fresh whole cranberries
    2 Tbsp. dark brown sugar
    2 tsp. cornstarch mixed with 2 Tbsp. water

Cut ham steaks into 8 equal portions. Lightly coat skillet with vegetable oil spray. Heat ham on both sides until browned. Transfer to large platter.

Add cider, bourbon, vinegar, onion, and the 1 c. cranberries to skillet, and heat until liquid is reduced by half. Add the other ½ c. cranberries.

Stir in brown sugar and cornstarch-water mixture and cook until sauce is thickened. Pour cranberry sauce over ham.

YIELD: 8 servings

Each serving: 218.1 calories, 6.3 g fat (26.0% calories from fat), 2.1 g saturated fat, 0.6 g polyunsaturated fat, 3.0 g monounsaturated fat, 60 mg cholesterol, 15.6 g carbohydrate, 23.8 g protein, 683 mg sodium

EXCHANGES: 3 lean meats; 1 fruit

Honey-Mustard Pork Medallions

◆

Serve these pork medallions with boiled parsleyed potatoes, bread, and a salad, and no one will ever guess that this meal was so simple!

  1½ lb. boneless pork tenderloin cut into six ½-inch-thick
     medallions, all visible fat removed
  4 Tbsp. mild brown mustard, or 2 Tbsp. spicy, robust
     brown mustard
  4 Tbsp. clover honey
  Optional: 2 Tbsp. dry red wine
  ¾ c. water
  Optional: 1 Tbsp. cornstarch mixed with 1 Tbsp. water

Lightly coat nonstick skillet with vegetable oil spray. Add pork medallions and brown on both sides, adding small amounts of water, a tablespoon at a time, if needed to prevent sticking. When pork is no longer pink inside, transfer to serving dish. Combine mustard, honey, red wine if desired, and water in skillet. Cook until sauce is reduced by about half. If you'd like a thicker sauce, add cornstarch-water mixture and cook until thickened. Serve medallions hot, topped with sauce.

YIELD: 6 servings

Each serving: 241 calories, 5.7 g fat (21.3% calories from fat), 1.9 g saturated fat, 0.7 g polyunsaturated fat, 2.5 g monounsaturated fat, 105 mg cholesterol, 12.5 g carbohydrate, 32.9 g protein, 140 mg sodium

EXCHANGES: 4 extra-lean meats; 1 fruit

Kielbasa and Cabbage

Sausage of any kind is generally very high in fat, but some of the new turkey sausages are much leaner than the original versions, and this recipe uses only a small amount. Be sure to read the label. Healthy Choice, for example, has a kielbasa-type sausage that contains only one gram of fat per ounce. Serve this dish with fruit, whole grain bread, and boiled potatoes (or add cooked potatoes to the prepared dish) for a hearty country meal.

½ lb. low-fat kielbasa-style turkey sausage
8 c. shredded cabbage (approx. ½ large head)

¼ c. plus ¼ c. chicken broth or bouillon
Optional: 1 Tbsp. Worcestershire sauce
⅛ tsp. ground black pepper
¼ t. caraway seeds

Place sausage, cabbage, and ¼ c. broth in nonstick skillet. Cook over high heat, stirring constantly. Add the additional broth as needed to keep cabbage from sticking. When cabbage is crisp-tender, let broth evaporate, and stir in Worcestershire sauce, if desired, pepper, and caraway seeds.

YIELD: 6 servings

Each serving: 77 calories, 2.1 g fat (24.2% calories from fat), 0.7 g saturated fat, 0.3 g polyunsaturated fat, 1.0 g monounsaturated fat, 11 mg cholesterol, 5.6 g carbohydrate, 9.8 g protein, 510 mg sodium

EXCHANGES: 1 lean meat; 1 vegetable

MEATLESS MAIN DISHES

Pasta with Fresh Basil Tomato Sauce

——◆——

This dish is served with a nice light tomato sauce that's not at all heavy or overworked. Adjust the seasonings to your taste, adding more garlic, onion, fresh basil, salt, or black pepper to please your palate. You can use two teaspoons of dried crushed basil in place of fresh basil, if necessary, but the fresh basil is worth searching for.

1 can (28 oz.) crushed tomatoes with puree
¼ c. chopped yellow onion
1 clove garlic, pressed
⅛ tsp. ground black pepper
6 large fresh basil leaves, chopped
Optional: ½ tsp. salt
Optional: 1 tsp. sugar
8 oz. pasta, cooked
6 Tbsp. freshly grated Parmesan or Romano cheese
6 Tbsp. sliced black olives

Heat tomatoes, onion, garlic, and pepper in large pot, stirring occasionally, until tomatoes start to bubble. Immediately reduce heat, and cook 30–45 minutes, until mixture thickens to good sauce consistency. Add basil, taste sauce, and add salt, sugar, and additional pepper if desired. If sauce starts to pop during cooking, cover pan immediately and reduce heat further. Often the popping means that the sauce is thick enough.

Serve sauce over pasta. Sprinkle 1 Tbsp. cheese and 1 Tbsp. sliced black olives over top of each serving.

YIELD: 6 servings

Each serving: 189 calories, 3.0 g fat (14.3% calories from fat), 0.9 g saturated fat, 0.2 g polyunsaturated fat, 0.4 g monounsaturated fat, 4 mg cholesterol, 33 g carbohydrate, 8 g protein, 384 mg sodium

EXCHANGES: 2 breads; ½ lean meat

Pasta with "Cream Sauce"

———◆———

This delicious recipe is nice when you're in the mood to enjoy pasta for its own sake, without many extras. Several subscribers have told me that this has become one of their favorite recipes.

1 Tbsp. olive oil
1 clove garlic, pressed
8 oz. pasta, cooked
½ c. evaporated skim milk
¼ tsp. salt
½ c. freshly grated Parmesan or Romano cheese
Optional: Freshly ground black pepper

Heat olive oil in large skillet. Add garlic and pasta, tossing to heat through. Add evaporated skim milk and salt, and heat 1–2 minutes, just until milk is thickened. Remove from heat immediately. Sprinkle with grated cheese and, if desired, freshly ground black pepper.

YIELD: 4 servings

Each serving: 291 calories, 7.0 g fat (21.6% calories from fat), 2.3 g saturated fat, 0.2 g polyunsaturated fat, 3.3 g

monounsaturated fat, 43 mg cholesterol, 43 g carbohydrate, 13 g protein, 348 mg sodium

EXCHANGES: 3 breads; ½ fat

Pasta and Broccoli

◆

I received this recipe from Mary Andrews of Grand Blanc, Michigan, who loves this dish because it is so easy and so fast. She makes it in large batches and then heats it up for lunch at work. One word of advice for brown baggers, though: Pack the cheese separately and add it *after* you reheat the pasta; otherwise you'll have a gooey mess.

> 8–9 oz. fresh pasta
> 2 c. fresh broccoli, cut up
> 1 clove garlic, pressed
> Ground black pepper to taste
> ½ Tbsp. olive oil
> Optional: ¼ tsp. salt
> Optional: ½ tsp. dried basil
> Optional: Ground red pepper to taste
> 3 Tbsp. grated Romano cheese

Cook pasta according to package directions. Add broccoli to pasta for last 1 minute of cooking time. Drain.

In large skillet, heat garlic and black pepper in olive oil over medium heat about 1 minute. Add drained pasta and broccoli. If desired, add salt, basil, and red pepper. Toss just until hot. Sprinkle ½ Tbsp. Romano cheese on each portion.

YIELD: 6 servings

Each serving: 102 calories, 2.8 g fat (24.6% calories from fat), 0.3 g saturated fat, 0.4 g polyunsaturated fat, 0.9 g monounsaturated fat, 18 mg cholesterol, 14.9 g carbohydrate, 5.7 g protein, 67.4 mg sodium

EXCHANGES: 1 bread; ½ meat; ½ vegetable

Quick and Easy Wintertime Linguine Primavera

──────◆──────

I developed this recipe after discovering Del Monte's new pasta-style tomatoes. Because the tomatoes already contain garlic, onion, and other seasonings, this is a really quick meal. If you cannot find the pasta-style product in your market, substitute Italian-style stewed tomatoes.

    10 mushrooms, sliced
    1 Tbsp. olive oil
    8 oz. linguine, cooked
    2 Tbsp. sliced black olives
    ¼ tsp. salt
    1 can (14½ oz.) Del Monte pasta-style stewed tomatoes,
        well drained
    ¼ c. freshly grated Parmesan cheese

In large skillet, sauté mushrooms in olive oil until just tender. Add cooked linguine and toss to coat well with oil. Add olives, salt, and tomatoes, and toss lightly until ingredients are well mixed. Sprinkle with cheese. Serve hot.

YIELD: 6 servings

Each serving: 199 calories, 5.2 g fat (23.6% calories from fat), 0.9 g saturated fat, 0.2 g polyunsaturated fat, 2.0 g monounsaturated fat, 3 mg cholesterol, 32 g carbohydrate, 6.6 g protein, 496 mg sodium

EXCHANGES: 2 breads; 1 vegetable; 1 fat

Linguine with Broccoli and Blue Cheese Sauce

The blue cheese adds a pleasantly surprising flavor to this linguine dish. Blue cheese is high in fat, but when used sparingly, as in this recipe, it can give a lot of flavor to a dish without contributing too much fat.

    4 c. broccoli florets
    2 cloves garlic, pressed
    ½ c. skim milk
    ⅛ tsp. ground black pepper, or more to taste
    8 oz. linguine, cooked
    3 oz. crumbled blue cheese

Lightly coat nonstick skillet with vegetable oil spray. Add broccoli and garlic, and sauté 1–2 minutes. Add milk, black pepper, and cooked linguine. When broccoli is tender, stir in blue cheese and serve at once.

YIELD: 6 servings

Each serving: 229 calories, 5.1 g fat (20.0% calories from fat), 2.9 g saturated fat, 0.4 g polyunsaturated fat, 1.2 g

monounsaturated fat, 11 mg cholesterol, 35.7 g carbohydrate, 12.7 g protein, 250 mg sodium

EXCHANGES: 2 breads; 1 vegetable; 1 meat

Rigatoni Bake

◆

Here's a simple Italian recipe that your children can prepare for the family and their friends. It's so easy that, if you don't watch out, you'll find yourself making it all the time! You can use penne instead of rigatoni, if you wish. Serve this casserole with hot Italian or French bread.

½ lb. rigatoni
2 c. low-salt canned tomato sauce
Optional: ¼ c. fresh basil or oregano, finely chopped
4 oz. feta cheese

Preheat oven to 350°F., and lightly coat casserole dish with vegetable oil.

Cook pasta according to package directions until al dente (cooked throughout but still somewhat firm); drain well. Transfer pasta to casserole dish. Pour tomato sauce evenly over pasta, and stir. Crumble cheese over all, and bake 20 minutes, or until cheese is browned and pasta and sauce are piping hot.

YIELD: 6 servings

Each serving: 203 calories, 4.6 g fat (20.4% calories from fat), 2.9 g saturated fat, 0.2 g polyunsaturated fat, 0.9 g monounsaturated fat, 17 mg cholesterol, 8.1 g protein, 32.7 g carbohydrate, 303 mg sodium

EXCHANGES: 2 breads; 1 vegetable; 1 fat

Vegetable Lasagna

———◆———

This has become one of my favorite dishes. The sauce can be assembled in just a few minutes. If you want to, make it up early and refrigerate it until you're ready to cook. Complement your lasagna with a salad, bread, and fruit, and you have a winner of a meal.

For many uses, fat-free cheeses do not compare with the low-fat cheeses, but they do work well in lasagna, especially when combined with part-skim (a low-fat) cheese. The fat content of low-fat cheese is lower than that of regular cheese, but when used in large amounts, as in this lasagna, it can still add a significant amount of fat and calories. That's why I use some fat-free cheese in this dish.

½ lb. lasagna noodles

Cheese Mixture:
8 oz. fat-free cottage cheese or ricotta cheese
4 oz. shredded fat-free mozzarella cheese
4 oz. shredded fat-free cheddar cheese
4 oz. shredded part-skim mozzarella cheese

Suggested Vegetables (use two or more):
1 large green pepper, sliced
1 large onion, sliced
½ lb. fresh mushrooms, sliced
1 pkg. (12 oz.) frozen spinach, thawed and squeezed dry
1 can (14½ oz.) Del Monte pasta-style or Italian-style
    stewed tomatoes, drained

Sauce:
1 can (28 oz.) crushed tomatoes with puree
1½ tsp. dried basil, or more to taste

1 clove garlic, pressed
¼ tsp. ground black pepper
Optional: 1 tsp. sugar
Optional: 1 tsp. salt

Cook lasagna noodles according to package instructions. Drain, rinse, and set aside. Combine all cheeses in another bowl and set aside. Clean and slice vegetables.

Mix together all sauce ingredients until well combined. Adjust seasonings to taste.

Preheat oven to 350°F. and coat 9-by-11-inch baking pan with vegetable oil spray.

Spread small amount of sauce on bottom of baking pan. Lay three noodles over bottom of pan. Spread one-third of remaining sauce evenly over noodles. Top with half of vegetables and then one-third of cheese mixture. Repeat for next layer. For third (top) layer, add only noodles, remaining sauce, and cheese (no vegetables).

Bake 45 minutes, until lasagna in middle of pan is very hot. Remove from oven, and leave at room temperature 5–10 minutes before cutting. (If cut sooner, it may be runny.)

YIELD: 12 servings

Each serving: 213 calories, 2.6 g fat (11.0% calories from fat), 1.0 g saturated fat, 0.2 g polyunsaturated fat, 0.5 g monounsaturated fat, 15 mg cholesterol, 25 g carbohydrate, 21 g protein, 721 mg sodium

EXCHANGES: 1½ lean meat; 1 bread; 1 vegetable; 1 skim milk

Eggplant Parmigiana

◆

This recipe must be prepared in a good nonstick skillet. Do not add water for sautéing, as the eggplant will not hold its shape.

1 large eggplant, peeled and sliced ½ inch thick
2 c. homemade tomato sauce or fat-free canned
   spaghetti sauce
½ c. shredded low-fat mozzarella cheese
2 Tbsp. grated Romano cheese

Preheat oven to 425° F., and lightly coat nonstick skillet with vegetable oil spray.

Brown eggplant on both sides in skillet, and place slices in 10-inch square casserole pan. (You may need to brown them in two batches and form two layers in casserole.) Cover eggplant evenly with sauce, and then layer cheeses over the top. Bake 10–15 minutes, or until hot.

YIELD: 8 servings

Each serving: 65 calories, 2.0 g fat (27.6% calories from fat), 0.8 g saturated fat, 0.2 g polyunsaturated fat, 0.4 g monounsaturated fat, 6 mg cholesterol, 9.4 g carbohydrate, 3.7 g protein, 66 mg sodium

EXCHANGES: 2 vegetables; ½ fat

Spicy Low-Fat Pizzas

———————◆———————

Pizza can be very low in fat, especially if you use cheese and topping sparingly. Try using a pizza stone or the slate (see the cooking tip that follows) if you want to make a truly sensational crust.

I sometimes make four small pizzas from this recipe. I top two or three of them with ordinary toppings and then experiment with the other one or two by trying more exotic combinations.

Crust:
1 recipe French Bread dough (page 183)
1 Tbsp. cornmeal

Sauce:
½ recipe Fresh Basil Tomato Sauce (page 117)

Toppings (use any of the following):
1 large green pepper, sliced
1 medium onion, thinly sliced
½ lb. fresh mushrooms, sliced
1 can (10 oz.) crushed pineapple, drained
½ lb. Canadian bacon or lean ham, chopped
½ lb. extra-lean ground beef
½ lb. low-fat Italian-style turkey sausage
½ lb. small shrimp, peeled and cooked
½ lb. turkey bacon, cooked and cut into small pieces

Cheese Topping:
6 oz. shredded fat-free mozzarella cheese
4 oz. shredded part-skim mozzarella cheese

Cut dough in half for two large pizzas. Roll dough out onto floured work surface until ¼-inch thick (dough will double in thickness as it cooks). If dough keeps shrinking, let it rest about 5 minutes and then try rolling it again.

Preheat oven to 500°F. Coat pizza pans with vegetable oil spray, sprinkle pan bottoms with cornmeal, and then place dough in pans, pulling it to fit. Bake the dough, untopped, about 5 minutes, or until it begins to brown slightly.

Remove the crusts from oven. Spread tomato sauce over crust, and sprinkle with your choice of topping and then with the cheese mixture. Bake just until cheese begins to bubble, crust is cooked, and all toppings are hot.

Y I E L D : **2 large pizzas (16 servings)**

Each serving of cheese pizza (⅛ large pizza): 170 calories, 2.9 g fat (15.4% calories from fat), 1.4 g saturated fat, 0.2 g polyunsaturated fat, 0.7 g monounsaturated fat, 9 mg cholesterol, 28 g carbohydrate, 7 g protein, 271 mg sodium

E X C H A N G E S : **1 bread, 1 vegetable, ½ skim milk, 1 fat**

Tip: The secret to an extra-crispy crust lies in baking your pizza or bread on a pizza or bread stone. These stones, or tiles, are available at kitchen specialty shops, but a less expensive alternative is a sheet of slate from a hardware store or stone quarry.

Before going out to buy your slate, carefully measure your oven rack. Then look for a sheet that is slightly smaller than your rack. Be sure to choose one that you can lift comfortably! Bring it home, and scrub it well with a heavy-duty scrub brush and soap and water. Sterilize the slate by placing it in your oven at 500–550°F for 30 minutes.

Each time you use the slate, place it on the top rack, and preheat it for at least 15 minutes before placing the food directly on it. (Do not use a pan.) A bread peel, which looks like a large wooden paddle, dusted with cornmeal, is used for transferring the bread or pizza into and out of the oven.

Pesto Pizza

◆

For a delightful change from ordinary pizza, try this pesto pizza. To make the crust, follow the recipe for making French bread dough, except use ½ of all of the ingredients. Follow the same procedure.

See the tip for baking extra-crispy crusts which follows the preceding recipe.

½ recipe French Bread dough (page 183)
1 Tbsp. cornmeal
¼ c. pesto
1 large green pepper, sliced
1 medium onion, thinly sliced
1 medium tomato, thinly sliced

Roll dough out onto floured work surface until ¼-inch thick (dough will double in thickness as it cooks). If dough keeps shrinking, let it rest about 5 minutes and then try rolling it again.

Preheat oven to 500°F. Coat one pizza pan with vegetable oil spray, sprinkle pan bottom with cornmeal, and then place dough in pan, pulling it to fit. Bake the dough, untopped, about 5–10 minutes, or until it begins to brown slightly.

Remove pan from oven. Spread the pesto over the crust. Add the sliced vegetables, and place back in oven. Bake for about 5 minutes, or until crust has finished cooking.

Y I E L D : **1 large pizza (8 servings)**

Each serving (⅛ pizza): 108 calories, 3.5 g fat (29.2% calories from fat), 0.7 g saturated fat, 0.2 g polyunsaturated fat, 2.3 g monounsaturated fat, 0 mg cholesterol, 15.8 g carbohydrate, 3.4 g protein, 196 mg sodium

E X C H A N G E S : **¾ bread, 1 vegetable, ½ fat**

English Muffin Pizzas

◆

English muffins make a good pizza crust when you're in a rush. They're also great for afterschool snacks, because most children enjoy making them by themselves.

```
3 English muffins, split
½ c. tomato or spaghetti sauce
Optional: ½ c. sliced raw vegetables
½ c. shredded part-skim mozzarella cheese
```

Preheat oven to 400°F. Lay English muffin halves on a baking sheet. Spread the tomato or spaghetti sauce over the muffins, and top with sliced vegetables and shredded cheese. Bake for 5–10 minutes, or until cheese has melted but has not begun to brown.

YIELD: 6 mini-pizzas

Each serving (one pizza): 117 calories, 2.2 g fat (16.9% calories from fat), 1.1 g saturated fat, 0.2 g polyunsaturated fat, 0.6 g monounsaturated fat, 5 mg cholesterol, 15.3 g carbohydrate, 5.5 g protein, 363 mg sodium

EXCHANGES: 1 lean meat, 1 bread

Easy California White Pita Pizzas

◆

This simple recipe is perfect for days when you have no time to cook. Pita bread makes a wonderfully crisp crust and cooks fast. Feel free to add tomato sauce or other ingredients, if you wish.

For each pizza:
1 small pita pocket, 6–7 inches across
¼ clove garlic, sliced
Sliced red or green peppers, onions, mushrooms, and
    tomato chunks (fresh or canned)
1 oz. shredded part-skim mozzarella cheese

Preheat oven to 450°F. Lay pita bread on baking sheet. Rub surface of bread with garlic, and either leave or discard, depending on how much garlic flavor you want. Top with sliced vegetables and cheese.

Bake 5–10 minutes, or until cheese is melted and vegetables are cooked to taste.

YIELD: 1 small pizza

Each pizza: 238 calories, 5.2 g fat (19.7% calories from fat), 3.0 g saturated fat, 0.5 g polyunsaturated fat, 1.3 g

monounsaturated fat, 16 mg cholesterol, 34.4 g carbohydrate,
12.3 g protein, 454 mg sodium

EXCHANGES: 2 bread; 1 vegetable; 1 meat

All-American Macaroni and Cheese

This recipe received an A+ from a subscriber who had tried
other low-fat macaroni and cheese recipes and found them to
be either rubbery or tasteless.

When I make this dish for my family, I sometimes add raw
chopped onion and red peppers to half of it. My husband and
I enjoy that part, while our children eat the plain half.

8 oz. (2 c.) uncooked elbow macaroni
2 Tbsp. all-purpose flour
1 c. skim milk
½ tsp. salt
1 tsp. prepared mustard
½ tsp. Worcestershire sauce
2 oz. (½ c.) plus ½ oz. shredded low-fat shredded
    cheddar cheese
½ c. unseasoned fresh bread crumbs

Cook macaroni according to package instructions.
Drain well. In large saucepan, whisk flour into cold
skim milk until no lumps remain. Add salt and mustard, and heat, stirring constantly, until mixture begins
to bubble hard. Immediately remove pan from heat,
and stir in Worcestershire sauce, cheese, and drained
macaroni.

Preheat oven to 350°F. and lightly coat baking dish
with vegetable oil spray. Pour macaroni mixture into

dish, and top with bread crumbs. Bake 20–30 minutes, until piping hot.

YIELD: 8 servings

Each serving: 129 calories, 2.1 g fat (14.7% calories from fat), 1.0 g saturated fat, 0.0 g polyunsaturated fat, <0.1 g monounsaturated fat, 7 mg cholesterol, 20.8 g carbohydrate, 6.5 g protein, 259 mg sodium

EXCHANGES: 1 bread; ½ skim milk; ½ fat

Red Beans and Rice

It seems that every time I travel, I come home with a new favorite recipe. Before we visited New Orleans, I had never eaten red beans and rice, but now it is one of my quick and easy (and very low-fat) favorites. Pass the hot sauce, or Tabasco sauce, and let people add just the right amount of heat for their individual tastes.

2 c. chicken broth or stock
1 can (16 oz.) whole tomatoes with juice, well broken up
½ c. water
½ c. chopped onion
⅓ c. finely chopped green bell pepper
2–3 cloves garlic, pressed
½ tsp. salt (omit if broth contains salt)
½ c. water
1 Tbsp. Worcestershire sauce
1 tsp. dried crushed oregano
½ tsp. Tabasco sauce
¼ ground tsp. black pepper

2 cans (16 oz. each) red beans or kidney beans, drained
   and rinsed
1 c. tomato paste
3 c. hot cooked rice

Place all ingredients except beans, tomato paste, and
rice in large pot, and bring to a boil. Reduce heat to
medium, simmer 15 minutes or so, and add beans and
tomato paste. Taste and adjust seasonings. Serve over
hot rice.

YIELD: 6 servings

Each serving: 287 calories, 1.6 g fat (5.0% calories from
fat), 0.3 g saturated fat, 0.6 g polyunsaturated fat, 0.3 g
monounsaturated fat, <1 mg cholesterol, 57 g carbohydrate,
13.0 protein, 455 mg sodium

EXCHANGES: 3 breads; 2 vegetables.

Sweet Peppers Stuffed with Brown Rice

◆

Martha Jolkovski, a good friend of mine, created this recipe
using an overabundance of large sweet yellow peppers from
my brother's garden, but you can use green or red peppers
instead. Feel free to substitute white rice or barley for the
brown rice, if you like.

6 large yellow bell peppers
3 c. cooked brown rice
4 oz. fat-free cheddar cheese
2 oz. extra-sharp cheddar cheese
1 c. diced mushrooms

1 small onion, chopped
½ c. frozen corn
1 large tomato, diced
Optional: Salt and pepper to taste
3 Tbsp. shredded Romano cheese

Slice off tops of peppers, and remove seeds and membranes. Cut usable parts of tops into chunks.

Preheat oven to 375°F.

Toss all ingredients except Romano cheese together in large bowl. (Be sure to add pepper chunks.) If desired, add black pepper and salt to taste. Stuff mixture into peppers, packing lightly, and place them in baking dish. Add ½ inch water.

Bake 40 minutes, or until peppers are tender. If rice starts to dry out, cover dish with foil for rest of baking period. Sprinkle ½ Tbsp. Romano cheese on top of each, and serve hot.

YIELD: 6 servings

Each serving: 238 calories, 5.6 g fat (21.2% calories from fat), 2.1 g saturated fat, 0.4 g polyunsaturated fat, 1.0 g monounsaturated fat, 16 mg cholesterol, 38.1 g carbohydrate, 10.3 g protein, 426 mg sodium

EXCHANGES: 2 breads; 2 vegetables; 1 fat

Cheese Enchiladas with Red Chili Sauce

If you've never tried making homemade corn tortillas, you really should try sometime. It's not hard, and the flavor is wonderfully fresh. Instead of flour, I use masa harina (found near the cornmeal and flour in some supermarkets, made by the Quaker Oats Company. I follow the instructions on the bag, except that I always add a bit extra water (1¼ to 1½ cup instead of 1 cup).

These enchiladas can be assembled fast and are quite a bit better than those served in most Mexican restaurants, especially when made with fresh tortillas!

Sauce:
2 c. beef broth, canned or homemade
2 Tbsp. all-purpose flour
3 Tbsp. chili powder
1 clove garlic, pressed
½ tsp. ground cumin
½ tsp. dried oregano
1 c. pureed tomatoes, canned or fresh

Enchiladas:
10 corn tortillas
2 c. low-fat cheddar cheese
1 medium onion, chopped
1 can (7 oz.) chopped green chilies

Garnish:
1 c. fat-free sour cream
2 Tbsp. chopped fresh cilantro or parsley

Whisk together broth, flour, and chili powder until all flour is dispersed in liquid. Add rest of sauce ingredients, and heat to boiling, stirring constantly. Reduce heat, and simmer while preparing rest of dish.

Preheat oven to 350°F. Coat bottom of baking dish with about ½ c. sauce. Heat tortillas thoroughly (20–30 seconds in bag in microwave or approximately 10 minutes wrapped in foil in 350°F. oven). Place one hot tortilla on work surface. Sprinkle about one-tenth of the cheese, onion, and green chilies down center, roll tortilla up, and place in baking dish. Repeat for all ten tortillas.

Pour sauce over tortillas and heat in oven 15–20 minutes, until hot throughout. Place two enchiladas on each plate, and top each with fat-free sour cream and chopped cilantro or parsley.

YIELD: 5 servings

Each serving (2 enchiladas): 311 calories, 10.3 g fat (29.9% calories from fat), 5.0 g saturated fat, 0.6 g polyunsaturated fat, 0.4 g monounsaturated fat, 33 mg cholesterol, 37.6 g carbohydrate, 21.8 g protein, 518 mg sodium

EXCHANGES: 2 meats; 2 breads; 1 vegetable

Southwestern Corn Bread Casserole
———◆———

This recipe is fun for corn bread lovers who also like spicy foods. It's best eaten right from the oven.

    1½ c. self-rising cornmeal
    4 oz. fat-free cheddar cheese, torn into pieces
    2 oz. extra-sharp cheddar cheese, shredded
    1½ c. fat-free sour cream

½ c. egg substitute
1 c. frozen corn
1 c. salsa
1 can (4 oz.) chopped green chilies
2 Tbsp. sugar
2 egg whites, beaten to soft peaks
1 large tomato, thinly sliced
Garnish: Fat-free sour cream

Preheat oven to 400°F. In large bowl, combine all ingredients except egg whites, tomato slices, and sour cream, stirring well. Gently fold in beaten egg whites just until well distributed throughout the mixture. Coat 9-inch square baking pan with vegetable oil spray, and add cornmeal mixture to pan. Bake about 25 minutes. Remove from oven and spread tomato slices over top. Continue baking until just set. Garnish each serving with dollop of fat-free sour cream.

YIELD: 9 servings

Each serving: 188 calories, 2.6 g fat, (12.3% calories from fat), 1.4 g saturated fat, 0.1 g polyunsaturated fat, 0.6 g monounsaturated fat, 8 mg cholesterol, 31.7 g carbohydrate, 9.8 g protein, 225 mg sodium

EXCHANGES: 1 bread; 1 skim milk; 1 vegetable; 1 fat

Eggplant Curry

◆

This is one of my favorite quick and easy eggplant recipes. Most eggplant recipes are high in fat, but this one omits all added fats. Add chunks of chicken breast along with the eggplant, if you wish.

Serve this curry over steamed rice.

6 c. peeled and cubed eggplant (1 large or 2 small
   eggplants)
½ tsp. salt
1 medium onion, coarsely chopped
3 cloves garlic, pressed
1 one-inch cube fresh ginger, minced
½ c. cilantro leaves, or 3 Tbsp. dried cilantro (coriander)
¼ c. water
1 tsp. ground turmeric
½ tsp. chili powder
½ tsp. ground cumin
¼ tsp. ground black pepper
¼ tsp. ground cinnamon
1 c. plain nonfat yogurt
1 c. canned crushed tomatoes, or 2 fresh tomatoes,
   diced
⅓ c. raisins

Cover eggplant with water, add the ½ tsp. salt, and stir. Let sit 1 hour. Drain, and wash off any remaining salt.

Lightly coat nonstick 1½ qt. saucepan with vegetable oil spray. Add eggplant, onion, garlic, ginger, cilantro, and water, and cook 5 minutes. When water evaporates, add rest of ingredients, and simmer until eggplant is tender and has begun to lose its shape.

YIELD: 6 servings

Each serving: 92 calories, 0.6 g fat (5.9% calories from fat), 0.1 g saturated fat, 0.2 g polyunsaturated fat, <0.1 g monounsaturated fat, <1 mg cholesterol, 20.2 g carbohydrate, 5.0 g protein, 218 mg sodium

EXCHANGES: 1 bread; 1 vegetable

Peppered Rice Pilaf

You'll love this colorful and tasty pilaf which is as simple as it is beautiful. Serve it either as a main dish or as a side dish. It can be prepared without the oil by "sautéing" the vegetables in water or vegetable broth, but the flavor and texture of the peppers is much improved by using a small amount of olive oil.

    1¼ c. uncooked brown rice
    2 c. boiling water
    1 Tbsp. olive oil
    2 *each*: large green, red, and yellow bell peppers, cored,
        seeded, and cut into 1-inch chunks
    1 medium onion, chopped
    2 cloves garlic, minced
    1 tsp. salt
    Optional: ⅛ tsp. ground black pepper

Add brown rice to boiling water. Reduce heat to low-medium, and cover. Cook until all water is absorbed

and rice is tender. Rinse in colander under cold water
to prevent clumping.

Heat olive oil until hot. Add remaining ingredients
to pan, and cook about 5 minutes, stirring to prevent
burning. Reduce heat to medium, and continue to
cook until peppers are softened. Add drained rice, and
heat until piping hot.

YIELD: 8 servings

Each serving: 115 calories, 2.4 g fat (18.6% calories from
fat), 0.2 g saturated fat, 0.2 g polyunsaturated fat, 1.3 g
monounsaturated fat, 0 mg cholesterol, 22.2 g carbohydrate,
2.8 g protein, 407 mg sodium

EXCHANGES: 1 bread; 1 vegetable; 1 fat

Fried Rice

———◆———

Fried rice is a wonderful "leftover" meal that can be adapted
to all tastes. Don't feel restricted to the vegetables suggested
here. Use whatever you happen to have on hand.

    1 large onion, chopped or cut into thin wedges
    2 cloves pressed garlic
    2 tsp. minced or grated fresh ginger
    1 c. shredded cabbage
    1 small carrot, shredded or cut into matchsticks
    1 c. mushrooms, thinly sliced
    3 Tbsp. soy sauce
    4 c. cooked rice
    2 scallions, cut into 1-inch lengths
    1 c. frozen green peas or fresh snow peas

Lightly coat large nonstick skillet with vegetable oil spray. Add onion, garlic, the 1 tsp. ginger, and the cabbage, carrot, and mushrooms, and sauté until vegetables are tender. Add ¼ c. or more water, if necessary, to prevent sticking.

Add soy sauce and rice, and toss until well mixed. Stir in scallions, peas and remaining 1 tsp. ginger, and cook, stirring, until mixture is hot. Serve at once.

YIELD: 8 servings

Each serving: 146 calories, 0.3 g fat (1.8% calories from fat), <0.1 g saturated fat, <0.1 g polyunsaturated fat, <0.1 g monounsaturated fat, 0 mg cholesterol, 31.3 g carbohydrate, 4.4 g protein, 400 mg sodium

EXCHANGES: 1½ breads; 1 vegetable

Indonesian Fried Rice

◆

For a fun change from Chinese fried rice, try this Indonesian version. It is delicious with or without the ground red pepper.

This tastes best when made with an Asian curry powder, but use McCormick or another supermarket brand if the Asian style isn't available in your area.

1 Tbsp. mild curry powder
½ tsp. ground turmeric
2 Tbsp. molasses
2 Tbsp. creamy peanut butter
Optional: ½ tsp. crushed red pepper
3 Tbsp. soy sauce
1 large onion, chopped or cut into thin wedges

2 cloves garlic, pressed
2 tsp. minced or grated fresh ginger
1 c. shredded cabbage
1 small carrot, shredded or cut into matchsticks
1 c. mushrooms, thinly sliced
4 c. cooked rice
2 scallions, cut into 1-inch lengths
1 c. frozen green peas or fresh snow peas

Combine the curry powder, turmeric, molasses, peanut butter, red pepper, and soy sauce in a small bowl. Set aside to use later.

Lightly coat a large nonstick skillet with vegetable oil spray. Add onion, garlic, ginger, cabbage, carrot, and mushrooms, and sauté until vegetables are tender. Add ¼ c. or more water, if necessary, to prevent sticking.

Add soy sauce mixture and rice, and toss until well-mixed. Stir in scallions and peas, and cook, stirring, until mixture is hot. Serve at once.

YIELD: 8 servings

Each serving: 184 calories, 2.4 g fat (11.7% calories from fat), 0.4 g saturated fat, 0.7 g polyunsaturated fat, 1.0 g monounsaturated fat, 0 mg cholesterol, 35.8 carbohydrate, 5.5 g protein, 425 mg sodium

EXCHANGES: 2 breads, 1 vegetable, ½ fat

Sesame Peppers

Here's a simple spicy stir-fry recipe. Feel free to add chicken breast strips, shrimp and/or scallops, or Sea Legs if you'd like.

The success of any stir-fried dish lies partly in the quality of the soy or tamari sauce used. Some have a good depth of flavor that can really enhance the dish while others do little more than add color and salt. Be willing to try different products before picking your favorite.

½ Tbsp. olive oil
Optional: Crushed or whole hot red peppers
2 *each*: large green, red, and yellow bell peppers, cored,
    seeded, and cut into 1-inch chunks
1 medium onion, chopped
2 cloves garlic, minced
1 tsp. grated fresh ginger
1 Tbsp. low-sodium tamari or soy sauce
1 Tbsp. toasted sesame seeds
2 c. hot steamed rice

Heat olive oil in large skillet. Add remaining ingredients, except sesame seeds and rice, to pan, stirring to prevent burning. Cook about 5 minutes, reduce heat to medium, and continue to cook until peppers are softened. Top with toasted sesame seeds, and serve mixture over hot steamed rice.

YIELD: **4 servings, with rice.**

Each serving: 150 calories, 3.7 g fat (22.2% calories from fat), 0.5 g saturated fat, 1.5 g polyunsaturated fat, 1.4 g

monounsaturated fat, 0 mg cholesterol, 23.4 g carbohydrate, 4.2 g protein, 450 mg sodium

EXCHANGES: 1 bread; 1 vegetable; 1 fat

SANDWICHES

Hawaiian Ham and Swiss Sandwich

———◆———

Here's a quick hot sandwich which combines three flavors that blend together nicely: ham, Swiss cheese, and pineapple. Use rye or pumpernickel rolls instead of kaisers, if you prefer. For best flavor and texture, serve this sandwich hot from the oven.

For each sandwich:
1 kaiser roll
2 oz. thinly sliced low-fat ham
1 slice (¾ oz.) low-fat Swiss cheese
1 pineapple slice
1 fresh parsley sprig
Optional: Lettuce for garnish

Preheat oven to 400°F. Slice roll in half, and lay halves side by side on baking sheet, cut side up. Place ham and pineapple slice on bottom half, and put cheese on top half of bun. Bake 7–10 minutes, until cheese is melted and pineapple and bread are hot.

Serve open-faced on plate with parsley sprig between the two halves. If desired, arrange lettuce around plate.

YIELD: 1 serving

Each sandwich: 275 calories, 8.1 g fat (26.5% calories from fat), 3.4 g saturated fat, 0.2 g polyunsaturated fat, 1.1 g monounsaturated fat, 27 mg cholesterol, 30 g carbohydrate, 20 g protein, 737 mg sodium

EXCHANGES: 2 breads; 2 meats; ½ fat

Hot Chinese Chicken Breast Sandwiches

My husband and I love this sandwich. It's best made with freshly cooked chicken breast, but try it, too, when you have leftover chicken breast that you need to use up.

For best flavor and texture, be sure that the chicken is warm and the buns are freshly toasted.

1 lb. boneless, skinless chicken breast, cooked and
    thinly sliced
4 sesame sandwich buns, halved and toasted
1 tsp. sesame oil
1 garlic clove, pressed
1 tsp. minced fresh ginger
1 Tbsp. low-sodium soy or tamari sauce
Shredded lettuce
Optional: Sliced tomato, onion rings, bean sprouts

Distribute chicken slices evenly among bottom halves of toasted buns. Combine sesame oil, garlic, ginger, and soy sauce, and spread mixture over chicken. Add lettuce and other vegetables as desired. Place top half on each bun and serve at once.

YIELD: 4 servings

Each sandwich: 328 calories, 7.4 g fat (20.3% calories from fat), 1.8 g saturated fat, 1.8 g polyunsaturated fat, 2.9 g monounsaturated fat, 96 mg cholesterol, 39.4 g protein, 22.8 g carbohydrate, 514 mg sodium

EXCHANGES: 5 extra-lean meats; 1½ breads

"Fried" Fish Sandwiches

_____◆_____

If you love the fish sandwiches served in fast-food restaurants, but you don't like the amount of fat they contain, try these fish sandwiches instead. Top them with this yogurt and dill sauce, or use a low-fat or fat-free tartar sauce from your supermarket instead.

1 recipe Sesame "Fried" Fish Squares (page 107)
4 sesame sandwich buns
¼ c. plain nonfat yogurt
1 tsp. dried dill
Optional: Pinch salt and pepper
Optional: Lettuce and sliced tomato

Lay one fish square on bottom half of each bun. Combine yogurt and dill. Add salt and pepper if desired, and spread some of the yogurt mixture on top of each fish square. Top with lettuce and sliced tomato, if desired. Replace top halves of buns and serve at once.

YIELD: 4 servings

Each sandwich: 295 calories, 5.0 g fat (15.3% calories from fat), 0.9 g saturated fat, 1.1 g polyunsaturated fat, 2.5 g

monounsaturated fat, 28 mg cholesterol, 33.2 g carbohydrate, 27.4 g protein, 468 mg sodium

EXCHANGES: 2 breads; 3 lean meats

Sandwich Roll-Ups

◆

Here's an opportunity to be creative. Use whatever lean meats you have on hand, but focus on loading these sandwiches up with thinly sliced raw vegetables. Serve them with fruit and a salad for a fast meal.

For each sandwich:
1 flour tortilla
1.5 oz. smoked turkey or other lean meat
1 sliced mushroom
2 thin slices tomato
2–3 thin slices onion
¼ c. alfalfa sprouts
1 Tbsp. fat-free ranch-style dressing

Lay tortilla flat, and lay meat and vegetables down center, avoiding the outer ½ inch or so. Sprinkle with the dressing, and roll up into fajita shape.

YIELD: 1 serving

Each roll-up: 192 calories, 3.1 g fat (14.5% calories from fat), 0.5 g saturated fat, 1.2 g polyunsaturated fat, 1.1 g monounsaturated fat, 35 mg cholesterol, 23.9 g carbohydrate, 16.9 g protein, 194 mg sodium

EXCHANGES: 1½ lean meats; 1 bread; 2 vegetables

VEGETABLES, GRAINS, AND SIDE DISHES

———◆———

I was lucky to grow up on a farm with a large garden and a mother who knew many wonderful ways to make all vegetables taste great. My mother froze and canned enough during the summer to last all year, so we were never without good vegetables.

I still love vegetables, but I've had to learn new ways of cooking some of them—new lower-fat methods that don't require the butter and pork seasoning that tasted so good back then. In this chapter you'll find lots of different methods of cooking vegetables, some of them incorporating techniques used in other ethnic cuisines. Be sure to check out the meatless recipes in the Main Dish chapter, as many of those recipes also use a lot of vegetables.

This section also includes grain recipes and side dishes, because many of them include vegetables and because people use them as they would use vegetables.

Nutrition experts encourage us to eat more vegetables and grains. Both are naturally very low in fat and include vitamins that are not readily available from the other food groups. Vegetables are a good source of vitamins A and C, natural antioxidants that seem to protect our bodies against heart disease, cancer, and some of the effects of aging. Grains are full of B-vitamins, complex carbohydrates, and both soluble and insoluble fiber.

Lemony Green Beans

◆

These green beans will add bright green color and mild flavor to any meal. Try this brown sugar and lemon combination on other vegetables, too.

1 lb. fresh green beans, ends snapped off but left long,
   or 1 package (20 oz.) frozen green beans
2 Tbsp. fresh lemon juice
1 Tbsp. brown sugar
Optional: ⅛ tsp. salt
Optional: Very thin lemon slices

Steam green beans just until tender. For bright green color, do not overcook. Drain, and toss with lemon juice and sugar. Add salt if you wish. Transfer to serving bowl. If desired, garnish with lemon slices.

YIELD: 8 servings

Each serving: 25 calories, 0 g fat (0% calories from fat), 0 g saturated fat, 0 g polyunsaturated fat, 0 g monounsaturated fat, 0 mg cholesterol, 6.1 g carbohydrate, 1.1 g protein, 4 mg sodium

EXCHANGES: 1 vegetable

Corn Pudding

———◆———

Corn pudding is one of my mother's specialties, a dish that she makes for large gatherings and holiday meals. Although usually served as a side dish, this can also be a great meatless main dish. For a crowd, double the recipe, and bake it in a larger pan.

1 can (16 oz.) whole kernel corn, *not* drained
1 c. evaporated skim milk mixed with ½ c. skim milk powder
½ c. egg substitute
2 Tbsp. sugar
1 Tbsp. all-purpose flour
Ground black pepper to taste

Preheat oven to 350°F., and lightly coat 8-inch-square baking pan with vegetable oil spray.

Whisk together all ingredients in large bowl, taking care to disperse the flour. Pour pudding into baking pan. Bake about 30 minutes, or just until set. Remove from oven, and let sit for at least 5 minutes before serving.

YIELD: 8 servings

Each serving: 122 calories, 0.7 g fat (5.2% calories from fat), 0.2 g saturated fat, 0.3 g polyunsaturated fat, 0.2 g monounsaturated fat, 3 mg cholesterol, 22.3 g carbohydrate, 8.4 g protein, 102 mg sodium

EXCHANGES: 1 bread; ½ skim milk

Two-Squash Casserole

———◆———

This is my mother's recipe—the first squash that my husband ever enjoyed eating. You can reduce the fat content of this dish even further by using the homemade bread crumbs instead of stuffing mix.

   2 large zucchini, cut into ½-inch-thick slices
   2 large yellow squash, cut into ½-inch-thick slices
   1 large onion, cut into thin wedges
   1 can (3½ oz.) sliced water chestnuts, drained
   1 c. fat-free sour cream
   Optional: ½ tsp. salt
   Optional: Ground black pepper
   1 c. crumb-type herb-seasoned stuffing mix or
      homemade bread crumbs

Steam squash and onion. Drain, and cool to room temperature. Toss with water chestnuts and sour cream. Add salt, if you wish. Pour into casserole dish and, if desired, sprinkle black pepper over surface. Top with stuffing mix.

To serve hot, heat in oven just until hot (sour cream may curdle if heated too long). This is tasty, too, eaten at room temperature.

YIELD: 10 servings

Each serving: 90 calories, 2.1 g fat (21% calories from fat), 0.4 g saturated fat, 0.6 g polyunsaturated fat, 0.8 g monounsaturated fat, <1 mg cholesterol, 14.5 g carbohydrate, 4.2 g protein, 138 mg sodium

EXCHANGES: 1½ vegetable; ½ bread; ½ fat

Grilled Vegetable Combo

◆

Don't be limited by the vegetables suggested here. Use your favorites or whatever you happen to have on hand. If you cannot find Crazy Jane's seasoned salt, use another seasoned salt or an herb mixture.

½ large green bell pepper, cored, seeded, and cut
  into chunks
1 small onion, quartered
1 medium yellow squash, sliced
1 medium tomato, coarsely chopped
10 whole mushrooms
1 tsp. Crazy Jane's seasoned salt

Preheat grill and lightly coat large sheet of aluminum foil with vegetable oil spray. Combine all ingredients on foil, fold foil around vegetables, and seal tightly. Grill on low to medium heat 15–20 minutes, turning at least once, until all vegetables are tender. Serve hot.

YIELD: 6 servings

Each serving: 20.8 calories, 0.2 g fat (8.7% calories from fat), <0.1 g saturated fat, 0.1 g polyunsaturated fat, <0.1 g monounsaturated fat, 0 mg cholesterol, 4.4 g carbohydrate, 1.0 g protein, 181 mg sodium

EXCHANGES: 1 vegetable

Portobello Mushrooms Topped with Vegetables and Feta Cheese

◆

Here is an unusual flavor combination that can serve as a main dish or as a vegetable course with meat. For a meatless meal, serve it with corn on the cob, fresh fruit, and French bread. Try to find mushrooms that are six or more inches in diameter, if possible.

The water from feta cheese can be great for seasoning sautéed vegetables or mixed with olive oil for a salad dressing. If you deplete the water in your container of feta cheese, add more before storing it in your refrigerator.

4 large Portobello mushrooms
4 large tomatoes, or 8 plum tomatoes, coarsely chopped
2 small zucchini, thinly sliced
1 medium onion, chopped
1 c. close-packed shredded fresh spinach
4–6 cloves garlic, pressed
2 Tbsp. chopped fresh parsley or 2 tsp. parsley flakes
2 Tbsp. chopped fresh basil, or 2 tsp. dried
1 Tbsp. chopped fresh oregano, or 1 tsp. dried
Optional: ½ tsp. salt
⅛ tsp. ground black pepper
½ c. water from feta cheese
6 tsp. crumbled feta cheese

Preheat broiler and coat large baking sheet with vegetable oil spray.

Gently pull stems from mushrooms, taking care not to break or tear tops. (Save stems for broth or other uses.) Wash any dirt from mushrooms, and dry them with towel. Place mushroom caps on baking sheet, gill side up.

Lightly coat nonstick skillet with vegetable oil spray. Place remaining ingredients except crumbled feta cheese in skillet, and sauté until tomatoes have lost their shape and most of the water has evaporated.

Top mushrooms with vegetable mixture, distributing it evenly among the mushrooms. Place 1½ tsp. crumbled feta cheese on top of the vegetable mixture on each mushroom cap, and slide baking sheet under broiler. Broil about 5 minutes, or until feta cheese browns. Serve hot.

YIELD: **4 servings**

Each serving: 110 calories, 2.7 g fat (22.1% calories from fat), 1.3 g saturated fat, 0.5 g polyunsaturated fat, 0.5 g monounsaturated fat, 7 mg cholesterol, 19.4 g carbohydrate, 6.4 g protein, 124 mg sodium

EXCHANGES: **2 vegetables; ½ skim milk; ½ fat**

Zucchini Fans

◆

1 small zucchini for each person
Italian-style seasoned salt or herb mixture

Wash zucchini and cut off stem. Create long, narrow fans by making slices along length of zucchini about ¼ inch apart, leaving at least ½ inch at one end uncut so that slices will all stay together. Sprinkle seasoning mix through slices and on top. Wrap zucchini individually in aluminum foil, and cook on grill, turning once, for 15 minutes, or until tender.

YIELD: 1 serving

Each serving: 18 calories, 0.2 g fat (10.0% calories from fat), 0 g saturated fat, 0 g polyunsaturated fat, 0 g monounsaturated fat, 0 mg cholesterol, 2.8 g carbohydrate, 1.6 g protein, 81 mg sodium

EXCHANGES: 1 vegetable

Whole Baked Apples

◆

These apples taste delicious with roast turkey or chicken as well as pork. Some people like to pour bourbon into the center of each apple before serving, but I like them just as they are here.

9 medium-sized red apples, washed and cored to within
  ½ or ¾ inch of the bottom
½ c. raisins
¾ c. dark brown sugar
½ tsp. ground cinnamon

Preheat oven to 350°F. Arrange apples in 9-inch-square baking dish. Place raisins in center of apples, distributing them evenly among the apples. Sprinkle brown sugar and cinnamon over all. Pour water into dish to depth of ½ inch. Bake 45–60 minutes, or until apples are soft. (Cooking time will depend on size and variety of apple.) Remove from oven, and let apples sit at least 20 minutes before serving.

YIELD: 9 servings

Each serving: 130 calories, 0.5 g fat (3.5% calories from fat), <0.1 g saturated fat, 0.1 g polyunsaturated fat, <0.1 g monounsaturated fat, 0 mg cholesterol, 33.9 carbohydrate, 0.5 g protein, 4 mg sodium

EXCHANGES: 2 fruits

"French Fried" Shoestring Potatoes

◆

I don't know anyone who doesn't like french fries. This recipe cuts the fat by baking them in the oven with only a small amount of oil. For variety, use a Cajun or spicy seasoning mix or garlic salt instead of the salt and pepper called for here.

    4 medium-large potatoes, peeled if desired
    2 tsp. vegetable oil
    Optional: ½ tsp. salt
    Optional: ⅛ tsp. ground black pepper

Preheat oven to 400°F. Lightly coat baking sheet with vegetable oil spray. Cut potatoes into thin shoestring sticks, and soak them in cold water.

Drain potatoes, and dry well between two dish towels. Toss well with oil and, if you wish, salt and pepper. Spread potatoes on baking sheet in one layer. Bake 20 minutes or until medium brown (time will depend on type and freshness of potatoes), turning once. Serve hot.

YIELD: 4 servings

Each serving: 136 calories, 2.4 g fat (15.9% calories from

fat), **0.4 g saturated fat, 1.4 g polyunsaturated fat, 0.5 g monounsaturated fat, 5 mg cholesterol, 27.0 g carbohydrate, 2.3 g protein, 7 mg sodium**

EXCHANGES: 2 breads; ½ fat

Indian Potatoes

◆

These potatoes make a wonderful accompaniment to tandoori chicken, but they can also be served as a meatless entrée.

6 canned plum tomatoes, mashed
1 medium onion, sliced
1–2 cloves garlic, pressed
¼ tsp. ground turmeric
¼ tsp. ground cumin, or more to taste
Pinch ground black pepper
6 small or 4 medium cooked new white potatoes, peeled
    or unpeeled, cut into ½-inch cubes

Coat large skillet with vegetable oil spray. Place all ingredients except potatoes in skillet, and cook until onions are tender. Add potatoes, and continue to cook until potatoes are hot. While cooking, stir frequently but gently, taking care not to break up potatoes. Serve hot or at room temperature.

YIELD: 6 servings

Each serving: 129 calories, 0.3 g fat (2.1% calories from fat), <0.1 g saturated fat, 0.1 g polyunsaturated fat, <0.1 g monounsaturated fat, 0 mg cholesterol, 28.7 g carbohydrate, 2.9 g protein, 72 mg sodium

EXCHANGES: 2 breads

Roasted Potato Wedges

———— ◆ ————

This is one of the first recipes that many students in my cooking classes decide to try at home. They love the flavor of these potatoes and the simplicity of preparation. Crush the sage leaves between your hands or in a mortar and pestle before adding them to the potatoes. This helps to release the natural oils and give more flavor.

    8 small white-skinned new potatoes, unpeeled and cut
        into wedges
    ½ Tbsp. olive oil
    ⅛ tsp. ground black pepper
    1 tsp. onion salt
    1 large clove garlic, pressed
    1 tsp. dried sage leaves, crushed

Preheat oven to 400°F. Combine all ingredients in large bowl. Lightly coat baking sheet with vegetable oil spray. Pour potatoes onto pan, and separate into one layer. Bake until browned and soft inside, about 20–25 minutes.

YIELD: 8 servings

Each serving: 118 calories, 1.0 g fat (7.6% calories from fat), 0.2 g saturated fat, 0.1 g polyunsaturated fat, 0.6 g monounsaturated fat, 0 mg cholesterol, 25.7 g carbohydrate, 2.4 g protein, 141 mg sodium

EXCHANGES: 1½ breads

Spiced Sweet Potato Slices

———◆———

This recipe is reminiscent of candied yams, but the spicy caramelized topping eliminates the need for butter. If possible, shop for sweet potatoes at a farmers market or food stand, as their sweet potatoes are often sweeter and more flavorful than the supermarket varieties.

    2 large sweet potatoes
    ¼ c. water
    ½ c. sugar
    1 tsp. ground cinnamon
    1 tsp. ground nutmeg
    1 tsp. ground ginger

Preheat oven to 350°F. Coat casserole dish with vegetable oil spray. Peel sweet potatoes and cut into ½-inch-thick slices. Place slices in single layer in casserole, and pour water into dish. Cover and bake until tender, about 30 minutes.

Remove dish from oven, and preheat broiler. Combine sugar and spices, and sprinkle over sweet potatoes. Place uncovered dish under the broiler, and cook 3–5 minutes or until sugar mixture bubbles and thickens on top of the potatoes. Serve at once.

YIELD: Approx. 12 two-slice servings

Each serving: 60 calories, 0 g fat (0% calories from fat), 0 g saturated fat, 0 g polyunsaturated fat, 0 g monounsaturated fat, 0 mg cholesterol, 14 g carbohydrate, 0.5 g protein, 3 mg sodium

EXCHANGES: ½ bread; ½ fruit

Mexican Rice

◆

For quicker preparation, substitute two cups of cooked rice for the water and raw rice in this recipe. To save even more time, if you're really in a hurry, substitute one cup of mild salsa for the tomato, green pepper, and chopped onion.

1 can (16 oz.) whole tomatoes, with juice
½ c. chopped green bell pepper
½ c. chopped onion
1 c. water
1 c. uncooked rice

Pour tomatoes and their juice into large saucepan, and break tomatoes into small pieces with whisk or your clean hands. Add pepper, onion, and water, and heat to a boil. Reduce heat to medium, and cook vegetables 5 minutes, or until peppers and onions begin to soften. Add rice, stir, and cover. Cook until water is absorbed, about 15 minutes.

YIELD: 6 servings

Each serving: 103 calories, 0.3 g fat (2.6% calories from fat), 0 g saturated fat, 0.1 g polyunsaturated fat, 0 g monounsaturated fat, 0 mg cholesterol, 23.4 g carbohydrate, 2.3 g protein, 191 mg sodium

EXCHANGES: 1 bread; 1 vegetable

Savory Bread Stuffing

◆

Although this herb-seasoned stuffing can be baked in a separate pan (using the larger amount of water), it tastes best
when cooked under the turkey breast, where it can absorb the
juices during baking. This recipe is mildly seasoned, but feel
free to add extra sage, thyme, and black pepper for a more
highly seasoned dressing.

    4 cups seasoned stuffing mix
    ½ c. chopped celery
    ½ c. chopped onion
    ⅔ can (14 oz.) Campbell's Healthy Request condensed
        cream of chicken soup, *no water added*
    ½ can water (⅔ can if cooking in baking dish)
    Optional: Salt, pepper, sage, and parsley flakes to taste

Toss together all ingredients in large bowl.

*If you're cooking the stuffing under the turkey
breast,* place stuffing in baking pan, and set turkey
on top. Push stuffing all up under breast, and cook
according to turkey instructions.

If you're cooking the stuffing in a separate dish,
place stuffing in 8-inch-square baking dish coated with
vegetable oil spray. Cover with lid or aluminum foil,
and bake 25–30 minutes until steaming hot.

YIELD : 10 servings

Each serving: 48 calories, 0.6 g fat (11.2% calories from
fat), 0.1 g saturated fat, 0.1 g polyunsaturated fat, 0.1 g
monounsaturated fat, 0 mg cholesterol, 9 g carbohydrate, 1 g
protein, 107 mg sodium

EXCHANGES : ½ bread

Basic Pilaf

◆

Here is a delicious basic pilaf, using just long-grain white rice. However, any grain may be substituted for the rice. If you want to combine grains that require different cooking times— such as wild or brown rice, bulgur, and millet—be sure to cook them separately and combine them just before serving. Cook the vegetables with just one of the grains or divide them among the different ones, and stir them into the finished pilaf.

1 c. chopped mushrooms
½ c. chopped celery
½ c. chopped onion
½ c. chopped red bell pepper
¼ c. water
¼ tsp. salt, or more to taste
1 tsp. lemon juice
1 c. uncooked long-grain or basmati rice
2 c. chicken broth
Optional: ¼ c. raisins
2 Tbsp. toasted sliced almonds
Optional: ½ large red bell pepper, cut into narrow strips
     and cooked in small amount water until tender

Place chopped vegetables, water, salt, and lemon juice in skillet, and "sauté" them until water has evaporated. Add rice, stir for 1 minute or so, and then add broth. When broth begins to boil, reduce heat to low, cover, and simmer until water is absorbed and rice is tender. (If all water evaporates before rice is tender, add more water ½ c. at a time until rice is cooked.) Toward end of cooking time, add raisins, if desired.

Serve hot, topped with almonds and, if you wish, red pepper strips.

YIELD: 8 servings as side dish or 4 servings as main dish

Each serving as side dish: 106 calories, 2.3 g fat (19.5% calories from fat), 0.3 g saturated fat, 0.5 g polyunsaturated fat, 1.4 g monounsaturated fat, <1 mg cholesterol, 18.4 g carbohydrate, 3.2 g protein, 170 mg sodium

EXCHANGES: 1 bread; ½ fat

Hominy Casserole

I loved hominy when I was growing up. The only problem was that I loved it fried in butter or with bacon, so I've had to find another way to enjoy it. My whole family enjoys this casserole, and it's fast, easy, and nutritious.

I like Manning's hominy, because it is a bit mashed and not liquidy. If your brand is packed in water, drain off part of the water and mash the hominy a bit or pulse it once or twice in the food processor before using it. If your local supermarkets do not have hominy, check the Latin American groceries.

2 cans (16–20 oz. each) hominy
3 scallions, chopped, both white and green parts
2 oz. lean ham, chopped
Optional: ⅛ tsp. ground black pepper
½ c. shredded low-fat cheddar cheese (5 g fat per oz.
   or less)

Combine hominy, scallions, and ham in nonstick skillet. Add black pepper if desired. "Sauté" until scallions are tender, and then top with cheese. Turn heat to low, and heat, covered, until serving time.

YIELD: 6 servings as main dish or 12 servings as side dish

Each serving: 117 calories, 2.4 g fat (18.5% calories from fat), 1.2 g saturated fat, <0.1 g polyunsaturated fat, 0.2 g monounsaturated fat, 9 mg cholesterol, 17.1 g carbohydrate, 6.9 g protein, 181 mg sodium

EXCHANGES: 1 meat; 1 bread

Barley-Mushroom Risotto

◆

Few people realize that risotto can be made with barley as well as with short-grain rice, and barley is much less expensive than arborio rice, an Italian short-grain rice. You can even make a risotto from steel-cut oats. It's good with garlic and rosemary. This version is my favorite, though. Add extra chopped vegetables if you wish.

½ plus 3 c. chicken or beef stock or broth
Up to 3 c. simmering water
½ lb. Cremini, Portobello, or button mushrooms, chopped
1 c. chopped onion
2 c. pearl barley
Optional: ¼ tsp. ground black pepper
Optional: Salt to taste

Heat broth to a simmer and keep it simmering. Place mushrooms and onions in separate pot. Add the ½ c. broth and "sauté" until onions are tender. Add barley, and stir well. Add extra broth from simmering pan, ½ c. at a time, whenever barley has absorbed all of the liquid. Cook barley, uncovered, about 45 minutes, stirring every few minutes, to develop the creamy "gravy." When all of the broth has been used, start using the water. When barley is tender, stop adding extra broth or water, and remove from heat. Taste and adjust seasonings.

Serve hot as accompaniment to chicken or lean beef, or serve as a main dish. Store in refrigerator. You may need to add water when you reheat the risotto, as the barley will continue to absorb liquid even as it sits.

YIELD: 10 servings

Each serving: 158.5 calories, 0.9 g fat (5.1% calories from fat), 0.1 g saturated fat, 0.1 g polyunsaturated fat, 0.2 g monounsaturated fat, <1 mg cholesterol, 33.4 carbohydrate, 5.2 g protein, 234 mg sodium

EXCHANGES: 2 breads

Cheesy Grits

Having been raised on a Virginia farm, I learned to eat grits at an early age, but it wasn't until I recently visited Charleston, South Carolina, that I learned to enjoy them. While there, I visited the Pinckney Café and Espresso and first tasted stone-ground grits. They're nothing at all like the supermarket variety that I grew up with.

You can order stone-ground grits from Hoppin' John's (a cookbook bookstore), 30 Pinckney Street, Charleston, SC

29401. The cost is $4.50 for a two-pound bag, plus shipping charges. By the way, "John" is really John Martin Taylor, the author of *Hoppin' John's LowCountry Cooking*. Check it out if you're interested in learning more about southern cooking.

Use good-quality grits from either yellow or white corn for this recipe.

1 c. grits
Optional: ¼ c. chopped onion or scallions
Optional: 1 Tbsp. chopped canned jalapeños
3½–4 c. boiling water
½ c. low-fat extra-sharp cheddar cheese
3–4 cheddar cheese shavings for garnish
Optional: ¼ tsp. salt

Slowly stir grits, onions, and jalapeños if using them, into 3½ c. boiling water. When grits begin to boil, reduce heat to medium, and continue to cook, stirring every minute or two, until thick and creamy, about 20 minutes. If you prefer thinner grits, add the extra ½ c. water. When the grits are cooked, add cheese and optional salt, and stir until cheese is melted. Serve hot, topped with shavings of cheese.

YIELD: 8 servings

Each serving: 75 calories, 1.4 g fat (16.8% calories from fat), 0.8 g saturated fat, <0.1 g polyunsaturated fat, <0.1 g monounsaturated fat, 5 mg cholesterol, 12.0 g carbohydrate, 3.6 g protein, 121 mg sodium

EXCHANGES: 1 bread

SALADS

◆

Salads are a favorite "health food" for many Americans. We eat them as appetizers, as main dishes, and as side dishes. Some of us even eat them for dessert.

Salads can be very nutritious. The food guide pyramid recommends that we eat at least 5 servings of fruits and vegetables each day, and eating salads can help us to meet this goal.

The most important tip to making a great salad is to use good quality ingredients. Insist on using fresh, crisp lettuce and fruits at their peak of ripeness. When your favorite greens or fruits aren't in season, try new ones.

Think of your menu when you select a salad recipe. Hearty entrées are usually best served with simply dressed green salads. Casual, informal meals might call for salads like coleslaw, potato salad, or a bean salad. Beautifully arranged salads can help to decorate a table at a buffet or large gathering.

Be aware, too, of whether you need to prepare the salad ahead of time or whether you have the time to dress and toss it at the last moment. When you're in a rush, choose a simple salad that doesn't have to be prepared ahead of time. If you're having guests, however, select a salad that you can prepare early and pull from the refrigerator when you're ready to serve it.

The salad recipes which follow range from lightly dressed assorted greens to a frozen fruit salad and a pineapple bowl. They are all low in fat but still delicious.

Tossed Romaine Salad

◆

It only seems appropriate that I include the recipe for my favorite everyday salad. This can hardly be called a recipe, though, because it's so informal and because it varies with whatever I happen to have on hand—part of a sweet red pepper, a bit of arugula, a handful of chopped herbs, a few croutons, and perhaps some sliced onion and tomato. But I do insist on a few things in my salad: fresh romaine lettuce—the lighter green inner leaves only; I throw away the tough, dark outer ones—a fruity olive oil, and a good balsamic vinegar.

If you use croutons, try the recipe below. The fat content of commercial croutons is often very high.

> ½ pound (approx.) romaine leaves, washed, dried, and
>   torn or cut into 1-inch pieces
> ⅛ tsp. salt, or less
> Freshly ground black pepper to taste
> 1 Tbsp. (approx.) balsamic vinegar
> 1–2 tsp. olive oil
> Optional: Homemade croutons
> Optional: Thinly sliced onion
> Optional: Vine-ripened or cherry tomatoes, arugula,
>   chopped fresh herbs, cucumber slices, red bell
>   pepper strips, or other fresh raw vegetables

Place lettuce in large bowl, and add salt, pepper, vinegar, and olive oil. Toss until lettuce is evenly coated. Add other ingredients as desired, and toss until well combined. Serve immediately.

YIELD: 4 servings

Each serving: 18 calories, 1.2 g fat (60% calories from fat),

0.2 g saturated fat, 0.2 g polyunsaturated fat, 0.8 g monounsaturated fat, 0 mg cholesterol, 1.4 g carbohydrate, 0.9 g protein, 58 mg sodium

EXCHANGES: ½ vegetable; ¼ fat

Croutons for Tossed Salad

———— ◆ ————

Whenever I have leftover French bread, I use it to make croutons. They are delicious. This recipe calls for either basil or oregano, but you may want to use both for more aromatic croutons.

4–6 c. bread cubes
1 Tbsp. olive oil
½–1 tsp. dried basil or oregano
1–2 garlic cloves, pressed
⅛ tsp. ground black pepper

Preheat oven to 325°F.

In large bowl, toss together all ingredients well. Spread on baking sheet in one layer. Bake 20 minutes, or just until croutons are crusty, stirring halfway through cooking period. Store in airtight container.

YIELD: 4–6 cups

Each 2 Tbsp. serving: approx. 14 calories, 0.6 g fat (38.6% calories from fat), <0.1 g saturated fat, <0.1 g polyunsaturated fat, 0.3 g monounsaturated fat, 0 mg cholesterol, 1.8 g carbohydrate, 0.4 g protein, 22 mg sodium

EXCHANGES: free

Lettuce and Orange Salad

———————◆———————

This is a bit similar to the romaine salad above, except that orange sections and sesame seeds give it a distinctive flavor. We especially enjoy this salad in the winter, when navel oranges are at their peak of flavor. You may want to use a whole red onion instead of just half.

```
1 lb. romaine lettuce, cleaned, dried, and cut into
    1-inch slices
4 medium-large navel oranges
½–1 medium red onion, thinly sliced and separated
    into rings
1 Tbsp. olive oil
2 tsp. balsamic vinegar
Optional: ⅛ tsp. salt
Freshly ground black pepper to taste
1 tsp. sesame seeds, lightly toasted
```

Place lettuce in large mixing bowl. Peel oranges and separate orange sections into bowl, squeezing juice from remaining membrane onto lettuce. Add remaining ingredients, and toss until well combined.

YIELD: **8 servings**

Each serving: 66 calories, 2.2 g fat (30% calories from fat), 0.3 g saturated fat, 0.4 g polyunsaturated fat, 1.4 g monounsaturated fat, 0 mg cholesterol, 11.1 g carbohydrate, 2.0 g protein, 5 mg sodium

EXCHANGES: **1 vegetable; ½ fruit; ½ fat**

Tomato Wedges with Sweet Basil Vinaigrette

---◆---

This salad is delicious, and it's always a winner when I serve it. Of course, it is best made with vine-ripened tomatoes, but I have made it in winter with drained canned tomatoes and had requests for the recipe.

2 medium-large tomatoes, cut into wedges
Optional: Sliced red onion, uncooked broccoli florets,
    cucumber slices
2 Tbsp. chopped fresh basil leaves, or ½ Tbsp. dried
    basil
1–2 tsp. sugar
1 Tbsp. cider vinegar
Optional: Ground black pepper to taste
Optional: Pinch salt

Place tomato wedges and other vegetables, if desired, in large mixing bowl. Add basil, sugar, and vinegar. Season with pepper and salt, if desired, and mix until well combined. Refrigerate up to 4 hours. Serve chilled.

YIELD: 6 servings

Each serving: 16 calories, 0.1 g fat (5.6% calories from fat), <0.1 g saturated fat, <0.1 g polyunsaturated fat, <0.1 g monounsaturated fat, 0 mg cholesterol, 3.7 g carbohydrate, 0.6 g protein, 5 mg sodium

EXCHANGES: ½ vegetable

Cucumber-Yogurt Salad

———◆———

This standard Indian salad is an excellent accompaniment to spicy main dishes such as tandoori chicken. Columbo and Dannon are my favorite brands of yogurt in this recipe.

2 c. thin cucumber slices
1 c. plain nonfat yogurt
⅛ tsp. black pepper
⅛ tsp. salt, or more to taste
Optional: ¼ tsp. ground cumin
Paprika

Combine all ingredients except paprika in large bowl and mix well. Refrigerate until serving time. Sprinkle with paprika before serving.

YIELD: 6 servings

Each serving: 26 calories, 0.1 g fat (5.9% calories from fat), <0.1 g saturated fat, <0.1 g polyunsaturated fat, <0.1 g monounsaturated fat, 0 mg cholesterol, 3.9 g carbohydrate, 2.4 g protein, 74 mg sodium

EXCHANGES: 1 vegetable

Old-Fashioned Coleslaw with Celery Seed Dressing

———◆———

6 c. shredded cabbage
½–¾ c. chopped sweet red pepper
2 Tbsp. shredded onion

¼ c. honey
3 Tbsp. cider vinegar
1 Tbsp. prepared mustard
½ tsp. celery seed
Pinch of ground black pepper
¼–½ c. fat-free sour cream

Combine all ingredients. Refrigerate until serving time.

YIELD: 8 servings

Each serving: 55 calories, 0.2 g fat (3.3% calories from fat), <0.1 g saturated fat, <0.1 g polyunsaturated fat, <0.1 g monounsaturated fat, <1 mg cholesterol, 12.9 g carbohydrate, 1.7 g protein, 44 mg sodium

EXCHANGES: 1 vegetable; 1 fruit

Molded Chunky Gazpacho

——◆——

Looking for a great make-ahead salad? This one might be for you. My mother gets lots of requests for this recipe.

2 envelopes unflavored gelatin
½ c. cool water
2 cans plain or herb-seasoned stewed tomatoes
½ c. chopped green pepper
½ c. chopped celery
½ c. chopped onion
Tabasco sauce to taste

In saucepan sprinkle gelatin over water, and let sit 2–3 minutes, until gelatin is softened. Heat water until gelatin dissolves, and then add remaining ingredients. Pour into 9-inch-square pan, and refrigerate until mixture congeals (at least 2–4 hours).

YIELD: 9 servings

Each serving: 34 calories, 0.2 g fat (5.3% calories from fat), <0.1 g saturated fat, 0.1 g polyunsaturated fat, <0.1 g monounsaturated fat, 0 mg cholesterol, 8.3 g carbohydrate, 1.2 g protein, 268 mg sodium

EXCHANGES: 1 vegetable

Pineapple Fruit Bowl

———◆———

This fruit bowl will decorate your table for any meal. The fruits listed are generally available, but feel free to use whatever other fresh fruits are available to you.

1 ripe fresh pineapple
2 bananas, peeled and cut into ¼-inch slices
1 c. seedless grapes
2 unpeeled apples, cored and chopped into ¾-inch
    chunks
½ c. fresh or frozen (thawed) raspberries, strawberries,
    or blueberries
Optional: Fresh mint leaves

Slice pineapple in half lengthwise using good-quality serrated bread or boning knife. With short-bladed utility or paring knife, cut out flesh of pineapple, leaving a shell approximately ¾ in. thick, and cut flesh into ¾-inch chunks.

In large bowl, combine 2 c. of the pineapple chunks (reserve rest for another use) with bananas, grapes, and apples. When well combined, add berries. Pour fruit mixture into pineapple shells, saving any extra fruit for refills. If desired, garnish with mint leaves.

Make-Ahead Note: Place pineapple shells in plastic bag and refrigerate. Combine pineapple chunks, grapes, and apples, and refrigerate in separate container. Just before serving, slice bananas and add to rest of fruit along with berries. Pour fruit mixture into pineapple shells.

YIELD: 10 servings

Each 1 c. serving: 51 calories, 0.3 g total fat (5.3% calories from fat), <0.1 g saturated fat, <0.1 g polyunsaturated fat, <0.1 g monounsaturated fat, 0 mg cholesterol, 13.2 g carbohydrate, 0.5 g protein, <1 mg sodium

EXCHANGES: 1 fruit

Fruited Cranberry Salad

Everyone I have ever served this to has wanted the recipe. I first ate a salad like this at a church potluck dinner, but could never find a recipe for it, so I had to devise my own. The red color and crunchy texture contrast beautifully with mildly flavored turkey, chicken, and pork.

For people on sugar-restricted diets, you can make this salad with sugar-free gelatin, leaving out the brown sugar and adding sugar substitute to taste.

1 c. boiling water
1 large pkg. raspberry-flavored gelatin
12 oz. fresh cranberries, coarsely ground
1 can mandarin oranges packed in light syrup, *not*
    drained, broken up into smaller pieces
1 can (20-oz.) crushed pineapple packed in juice, *not*
    drained
½ c. brown sugar, well packed
Lettuce leaves

In large bowl, add boiling water to gelatin, and stir until gelatin dissolves. Add cranberries, mandarin oranges with juice, pineapple with juice, and sugar, and stir until well combined.

Lightly coat salad mold or bundt pan with vegetable oil spray. Pour cranberry mixture into mold and refrigerate until solid. At serving time, invert salad onto plate lined with lettuce leaves. If salad will not fall from pan, dip pan in warm water 1–2 seconds and try again.

Y I E L D : **Approx. 14 servings**

Each ½ c. serving: **90 calories, 0 g fat (0% calories from fat), 0 g saturated fat, 0 g polyunsaturated fat, 0 g monounsaturated fat, 0 mg cholesterol, 22.3 g carbohydrate, 0.4 g protein, 14 mg sodium**

E X C H A N G E S : **2 fruits (1 fruit when made with sugar-free gelatin)**

Black Bean—Rice Salad

◆

You can make this salad spicier, if you wish, by adding more cumin and garlic. For best flavor, let the salad come to room temperature before serving.

1 can (16 oz.) cooked black beans, drained and rinsed
1 c. cooked brown rice
¼ c. chopped onion
¼ c. coarsely chopped green bell pepper
½ large tomato, cut into ½-inch cubes
1 small clove garlic, pressed
⅛ tsp. black pepper or more, to taste
1 Tbsp. lemon juice
1 Tbsp. apple juice
Optional: ¼ tsp. salt
Optional: ½ tsp. ground cumin
Optional: ½ Tbsp. canola oil

Combine all ingredients in large mixing bowl. Refrigerate until serving time.

YIELD: 6 servings

Each serving: 125 calories, 0.6 g fat (4.3% calories from fat), 0.1 g saturated fat, <0.1 g polyunsaturated fat, 0.1 g monounsaturated fat, 0 mg cholesterol, 24.5 g carbohydrate, 6.3 g protein, 74 mg sodium

EXCHANGES: 1½ breads; 1 vegetable

Note: If you add canola oil, fat content changes to 1.8 grams total fat per serving. Exchanges with canola oil: 1½ breads; 1 vegetable; ⅓ fat

Old-Fashioned Potato Salad

———◆———

Summer just doesn't seem like summer without potato salad. This is a very low-fat version of the potato salad my mother always made.

4 large or 6 medium new potatoes, peeled, cooked,
    and cubed
¼ c. chopped onions
½ c. chopped celery
4 boiled egg whites, chopped
Dressing:
¾ c. fat-free sour cream
10 bread-and-butter pickle slices, chopped
1½ Tbsp. pickle juice
⅛ tsp. ground black pepper
½ tsp. prepared mustard
1 tsp. salt
¼ tsp. celery seed
Lettuce leaves

Place potatoes, onions, celery, and chopped egg whites in large mixing bowl. Combine dressing ingredients, add to potato mixture, and toss until well combined. Refrigerate until serving time. Serve in bowl lined with lettuce.

YIELD: **8 servings**

Each ½ cup serving: 107 calories, 0.2 g fat (1.7% calories from fat), 0.1 g saturated fat, 0.1 g polyunsaturated fat, <0.1 g monounsaturated fat, 0 mg cholesterol, 24 g carbohydrate, 3.1 g protein, 206 mg sodium

EXCHANGES: **1½ breads**

Pasta Salad

◆

1 large tomato, chopped
¼ tsp. salt
2 Tbsp. chopped fresh basil, or 2 tsp. dried
1 Tbsp. chopped fresh oregano or 1 tsp. dried
2 cloves garlic, pressed
12 oz. spinach linguine or fettuccine
4 c. broccoli florets
½ c. chopped onion
½ c. grated Romano or Parmesan cheese
⅛ tsp. ground black pepper

Mix together the chopped tomato, salt, basil, oregano, and garlic, and set aside.

Cook linguine or fettuccine according to package instructions, adding broccoli to pot for last 1 minute of cooking. Drain noodles and broccoli, and transfer to large mixing bowl. Add tomato mixture, onion, cheese, and pepper. Adjust seasoning to taste. Serve immediately, or refrigerate until 30 minutes before serving. Tastes best if served at room temperature.

YIELD: 8 servings

Each serving: 106 calories, 2.2 g fat (18.7% calories from fat), 1.0 g saturated fat, 0.3 g polyunsaturated fat, 0.6 g monounsaturated fat, 14 mg cholesterol, 16.7 g carbohydrate, 7.4 g protein, 189 mg sodium

EXCHANGES: 1 bread; ½ vegetable; ½ meat

Couscous Salad

———— ◆ ————

This salad is quickly becoming a classic with many Americans. Try this oil-free version, too, with bulgur wheat for a chewier texture and different color.

Add some olive oil to this salad, if you wish, but use one with a lot of flavor. And remember that one teaspoon of any vegetable oil contains approximately 5 grams fat and 45 calories, so use it sparingly.

1 c. boiling water
1 c. couscous
1 c. chopped tomato or halved cherry tomatoes
1 c. chopped cucumber
⅔ c. chopped scallions, both white and green parts
1 clove garlic, pressed
1 can (16 oz.) garbanzo beans (chickpeas), drained
Optional: ¼ tsp. salt
Optional: ⅛ tsp. ground black pepper
Optional: 1 tsp. balsamic vinegar

In large bowl, pour boiling water over couscous. Cover bowl with plate, and set aside for at least 30 minutes. When grain is tender, fluff with fork and transfer to mixing bowl. Stir in remaining ingredients, adjusting seasonings to taste. Refrigerate until serving time.

YIELD: 4 servings

Each serving: 142 calories, 1.3 g fat (8.2% calories from fat), 0.1 g saturated fat, 0.5 g polyunsaturated fat, 0.2 g monounsaturated fat, 0 mg cholesterol, 27.8 g carbohydrate, 5.4 g protein, 183 mg sodium

EXCHANGES: 1½ breads; 1 vegetable

Tabbouleh

Here's another modern-day classic, also adapted from Middle Eastern cuisine. Once again, use olive oil if you wish, but add 5 grams fat for every teaspoon you stir in. Also feel free to add extra mint, but this is the amount that seems right to my taste.

> 2 c. boiling vegetable broth, chicken broth, or water
> ¾ c. bulgur wheat
> 2 c. chopped fresh parsley
> ½ c. chopped onion
> 1 clove garlic, pressed
> 2 Tbsp. finely chopped fresh mint leaves
> 2 Tbsp. fresh lemon juice
> ½ tsp. salt (omit if using salted broth)
> ½ tsp. ground black pepper
> 2 c. chopped ripe tomato
> Lettuce leaves

Pour boiling broth or water over bulgur, and set aside for at least 1 hour. Drain bulgur in sieve, pressing out any extra liquid. Add remaining ingredients except lettuce, mixing well. Adjust seasonings to taste. Refrigerate at least 1 hour to let flavors blend. Serve on bed of lettuce.

YIELD: 6 servings

Each serving: 137 calories, 1.6 g fat (10.5% calories from fat), 0.3 g saturated fat, 0.3 g polyunsaturated fat, 0.5 g monounsaturated fat, <1 mg cholesterol, 25.4 g carbohydrate, 7.1 g protein, 309 mg sodium

EXCHANGES: 2 vegetables; 1 bread; ½ fat

BREADS

Yeast Breads

Not many things in life are as satisfying as producing beautiful yeast bread. I make most of the bread our family eats, despite my hectic schedule. I've learned that the more you know about making yeast bread, the easier it is to fit it into your schedule.

Most breads today are made with active dry yeast, a granular yeast found in small packages in most grocery stores. It can be kept at room temperature, and is activated by softening it in warm water (110° F). (Water this temperature feels very warm but not hot to touch.) Water cooler than this won't activate the yeast, and water that is too hot can kill it.

All of the recipes in this section are made by the "Straight Dough Method." In this method, all ingredients are combined into a dough which is then kneaded and allowed to rise once or twice before being shaped. The dough is then given a final rising period and is then baked.

In most recipes, the dough will be left to rise in a greased bowl. You may use a heavy coating of vegetable oil spray, but I always rub a small amount of vegetable oil over the inside of the bowl. Place the dough in the bowl, rub it around a little, and turn it over, leaving a slightly oiled surface on the top of the dough. This light coating of oil, as well as covering the bowl with a cloth, helps to prevent the surface from drying out during the rising. Avoid getting the dough too hot or too cold while rising; too much heat can kill the yeast, and cold temperatures will prevent the dough from rising. If your stove has a pilot light, let the dough rise in the oven with the oven turned off.

I always make more bread than we can eat in one meal. I undercook bread that I intend to reheat later; I cook it to the doneness of "bake and serve" bread (cooked inside but not browned on the outside). To reheat, I place it in a hot oven (400°F or so) for 5–10 minutes. See individual recipes for instructions on how to reheat specific breads.

It takes practice to learn when bread is properly cooked. Rolls are cooked when they are medium brown and cooked throughout; check by separating two of them gently to see if the dough is cooked in between the rolls. Loaves are done when you remove them from the pan and they sound hollow when you thump them on the bottom. Never cut into a hot loaf of bread: it will be gummy and you can mash the loaf that way. Loaves slice best with a serrated bread knife.

This section includes recipes for several basic yeast breads—for dinner rolls, French bread, and whole wheat loaf bread as well as for soft pretzels and a yeasted nut ring. They are all fun to make and delicious.

French Bread

◆

Maybe you could say that I'm a fanatic about good homemade bread. If there is one recipe that I especially love sharing, this one is it. It is both simple and delicious, and it tastes good for three or four days when reheated. Leftovers make delicious croutons and bread pudding.

This recipe makes only one loaf (perfect for the size of my

food processor), but you can double, triple, or even quadruple the recipe when you want a larger yield.

Knead this dough by hand, if you wish, or in a mixer or food processor. I often use a food processor when I demonstrate French bread–baking to groups, because people are always so amazed at how easy it is to make and how delicious it tastes! You need a mixer or food processor with a strong motor, though. Stop if the machine begins to overheat, and finish kneading by hand. (See any basic cookbook for instructions on how to knead by hand.)

If you plan to make French bread regularly, I heartily suggest that you buy special baguette pans. They cook beautifully and allow you to produce well-shaped loaves with little effort, even if you have a minimum of experience. Keep a spray bottle filled with water on hand to spray the loaves before placing them in the oven.

1 tsp. or ½ pkg. active dry yeast
1 tsp. salt
1 c. water, slightly warm
2 c. plus ½ c. unsifted bread flour
1–2 tsp. vegetable oil

Place yeast, salt, water, and the 2 c. flour in large bowl. Knead 10 minutes by hand or in mixer with dough hook attachment, or 40 seconds in food processor. Add more flour, a small amount at a time, if dough is wet or too sticky. Before hand kneading, dust work surface with flour to keep dough from sticking. Dough should be smooth and soft at end of kneading period.

Grease bowl with oil. Place dough in bowl and turn it over so the oiled side faces upward. Cover bowl and dough with cloth, and leave in a warm place to rise until doubled in size (about 1 hour).

Punch dough down, and shape it into long loaf about 2 inches in diameter. Place in baguette pan or on baking sheet lightly coated with vegetable oil spray. Cover with cloth, and set aside until once again doubled in bulk (about 30 minutes).

Preheat oven to 400°F. Spray loaves with water from spray bottle. Place bread in oven, uncovered, and immediately reduce temperature to 350°F. Bake 30 minutes, or until bread is browned and feels crusty when squeezed.

To reheat: Place, uncovered, in 400–450°F. oven for 5–10 minutes, or until hot and crusty.

Y I E L D : 12 slices.

Each slice: 79 calories, 0.2 g fat (2.3% calories from fat), 0 g saturated fat, 0 g polyunsaturated fat, 0 g monounsaturated fat, 0 mg cholesterol, 16.5 g carbohydrate, 2.4 g protein, 178 mg sodium

E X C H A N G E S : 1 bread

VARIATION: For Tomato-Herb Bread, follow the French bread recipe above, but substitute ½ c. crushed tomatoes with puree for ½ c. of the water. Add ¼ tsp. dried oregano and/or other herbs before kneading, if you wish.

Y I E L D : 12 slices

Each slice: 84 calories, 0.3 g fat (3.2% calories from fat), <0.1 g saturated fat, <0.1 g polyunsaturated fat, <0.1 g monounsaturated fat, 0 mg cholesterol, 17.6 g carbohydrate, 2.6 g protein, 180 mg sodium

E X C H A N G E S : 1 bread

Old-Fashioned Dinner Rolls

◆

This is the dinner roll recipe that my grandmother taught me when I was a child. I still use it every year as a base for the sweet yeast breads I serve at Christmas dinner.

2 pkg. active dry yeast
2 c. warm water
½ c. skim milk powder
¼ c. sugar
1½ tsp. salt
2 Tbsp. vegetable oil
5½ c. bread flour

Add yeast to warm water along with skim milk powder, sugar, salt, and oil. Stir in flour until dough leaves sides of bowl. Turn dough out onto floured work surface and knead 10 minutes, or until dough is smooth and soft. Add small amounts of flour to work surface as needed to prevent dough from sticking during kneading.

Place dough in lightly oiled bowl, and turn so that oiled side faces up. Cover bowl with dish towel, and let dough rise until doubled (about 1 hour).

Lightly coat three cake pans with vegetable oil spray. Punch dough down with fist. Divide into balls about 1½ inches in diameter, and place in cake pans. Cover with dish towel, and let rise until once again doubled in bulk (about 30 minutes).

Preheat oven to 350°F. Bake rolls, uncovered, 30 minutes, or until lightly browned and cooked through.

YIELD: Approx. 36 rolls

Each roll: 81 calories, 0.9 g fat (10% calories from fat), 0.1 g saturated fat, 0.4 g polyunsaturated fat, 0.2 g mono-unsaturated fat, 2 mg cholesterol, 15.4 g carbohydrate, 2.3 g protein, 94 mg sodium

EXCHANGES: 1 bread

Whole Wheat Loaf Bread

I have always enjoyed good whole wheat bread, but it can be tricky to make and often is good only on the first day. Some whole wheat breads are also quite a bit higher in fat than you would expect.

Here's an oil-free recipe that is reliable and easy to make. I use some unbleached bread flour to improve the texture of the bread, and I add one egg to improve its "keeping" quality and give it a fine texture.

    1 pkg. active dry yeast
    2 Tbsp. brown sugar
    1½ c. warm water
    2½ c. whole wheat flour
    1 c. plus ½ c. bread flour
    ½ c. skim milk powder
    1½ tsp. salt
    1 egg or equivalent egg substitute
    Optional: 1 lightly beaten egg white

Stir yeast and brown sugar into warm water, and set aside about 5 minutes. In large mixing bowl, stir together the whole wheat flour, 1 c. of the bread flour, the skim milk powder, and the salt. Pour yeast mixture into flour mixture. Add egg, and mix until dough is all moistened. Dust work surface with ¼ c. of the remaining bread flour, turn dough out onto flour, and pour last ¼ c. bread flour on top of dough. Knead 10 minutes, or until dough is smooth and elastic. Add more flour, a tablespoon at a time, as necessary to prevent sticking, but be careful not to add too much so as to avoid making a dry loaf.

Lightly coat large mixing bowl with vegetable oil spray. Place dough in bowl, and spray vegetable oil lightly over top of dough. Cover bowl with towel, and set in warm place to rise until doubled in bulk (1 to 1½ hours).

Punch dough down, and pat into rectangular shape. Lightly coat 9½-by-5½-inch loaf pan with vegetable oil spray, and place dough in pan, pressing the dough so it touches all edges of the pan. Let rise again until doubled in volume (45 to 60 minutes).

Preheat oven to 350°F. For a shiny crust, brush egg white over top of loaf. Bake 35–40 minutes, until loaf is medium to dark brown on top and sounds hollow when turned out of pan and thumped on bottom.

Cool bread to room temperature on rack, or serve warm. Store in plastic bag.

Y I E L D : 1 loaf (approx. 20 slices)

Each slice: 103 calories, 0.7 g fat (6.1% calories from fat), 0.1 g saturated fat, <0.1 g polyunsaturated fat, 0.1 g monounsaturated fat, 14 mg cholesterol, 20.3 g carbohydrate, 4.4 g protein, 181 mg sodium

E X C H A N G E S : 1½ breads

Quick Soft Pretzels

◆

Pretzel making used to take several hours, but here's a recipe that streamlines the process to less than one hour. It requires no rising period and eliminates the need to boil the pretzels before baking them to give them a tough, chewy texture. For best results, be sure to cover the baking sheets with aluminum foil, because that's what gives the pretzels the steam they need for their tough texture.

1 pkg. (or 2¼ tsp.) active dry yeast
1½ c. warm water
½ tsp. salt
½ tsp. baking soda
3½ c. all-purpose flour
1 egg yolk mixed with 1 Tbsp. water
Optional: coarse salt

Preheat oven to 425°F., and lightly coat two baking sheets with vegetable oil spray. In large bowl, dissolve yeast in warm water, and set aside for 5 minutes. Add salt, baking soda, and flour, and stir until flour is incorporated.

Turn dough out onto lightly floured work surface, and knead 10 minutes. Cut dough into 4 equal parts, and then cut each quarter into 3 pieces, for a total of 12 sections. Roll each piece of dough into a rope about 16 inches long, and then twist it into a pretzel shape, pinching it together at points where dough overlaps. Place pretzel on baking sheet. Repeat with remaining pieces of dough. When all pretzels are formed, brush egg and water mixture on each, and top with coarse salt, if desired.

Cover baking sheets tightly with foil, trying not to let foil touch pretzels. Bake 10 minutes. Remove foil, and continue baking 5–10 minutes longer, depending on crispiness desired. (Shorter baking period yields very soft pretzels, and longer period produces crispier ones.)

YIELD: 12 large soft pretzels

Each pretzel: 127 calories, 0.6 g fat (4.2% calories from fat), <0.1 g saturated fat, <0.1 g polyunsaturated fat, 0.1 g monounsaturated fat, 11 mg cholesterol, 25.8 g carbohydrate, 3.9 g protein, 142 mg sodium (320 mg sodium if salted)

EXCHANGES: 1½ breads

Holiday Nut Ring

———————— ◆ ————————

This recipe makes two rings—one to eat immediately and another to freeze. When freezing rings, omit the glaze and add it just before serving.

To save myself the time and trouble of scalding the milk, I often substitute 1 cup water plus ¼ cup skim milk powder for the skim milk.

1 c. skim milk
2 pkg. active dry yeast
1 c. warm water
¼ c. sugar
1 tsp. salt
5½ c. bread flour
1 Tbsp. vegetable oil

Filling:
1 c. sugar
1 Tbsp. ground cinnamon
¼ c. toasted pecan pieces
½ c. currants, raisins, or other dried fruit

Glaze:
3 Tbsp. skim milk
1 c. confectioners' sugar

Heat the 1 c. milk just to boiling. Remove from heat, and set aside to cool until just warm to touch.

Dissolve yeast in warm water. Add sugar and salt. Add yeast mixture to cooled milk. Stir in 5 c. of the bread flour with wooden spoon, and stir until mixture leaves sides of bowl. Pour remaining ½ c. flour onto work surface, and turn dough out onto flour. Knead 10 minutes or until dough is smooth, adding extra flour to work surface if needed to prevent sticking.

Grease large bowl with oil. Place dough in bowl, and turn dough over so that oiled surface is on top. Cover bowl with towel, and set in warm place until doubled in bulk (about 1 hour).

Preheat oven to 350°F. and lightly coat two baking sheets or pizza pans with vegetable oil spray.

Punch dough down, and divide in half. Place one piece of dough on lightly floured work surface, and roll out into rectangle about 8 by 15 inches. Combine sugar and cinnamon, and sprinkle half of mixture evenly over entire surface of dough rectangle. Follow with half of the pecans and currants or raisins.

Roll up dough lengthwise into a roll 15 inches long. Pull ends together to form a ring, and press dough together firmly to seal. Make crosswise cuts ½ to ¾ inch apart from outer edge to within ½ inch of inner edge. Do *not* cut all the way through. When all the cuts are made, fan the pieces out, twisting and pulling each one slightly to make its edge slightly overlap the piece next to it. (All should overlap in same direction.) Now repeat process with remaining piece of dough to make second ring.

Bake 35–40 minutes, just until cooked through. Remove from oven, and cool 5 minutes.

Add milk to confectioners' sugar, using only enough milk to make a thick but slightly fluid glaze. Spread mixture over top of rings.

YIELD: Each ring, 14 servings

Each serving: 183 calories, 3.1 g fat (15.2% calories from fat), 0.3 g saturated fat, 0.7 g polyunsaturated fat, 1.8 g monounsaturated fat, <1 mg cholesterol, 36.5 g carbohydrate, 3.4 g protein, 85 mg sodium

EXCHANGES: 1 bread; 1½ fruits; ½ fat

QUICK BREADS

Quick Breads

◆

Breads which use baking powder and/or baking soda for leavening are called "quick breads." They don't require the lengthy kneading and rising time of yeast breads, because baking powder and baking soda start the rising process as soon as they are combined with moisture and heat.

Quick breads include most muffins, biscuits, and tea breads. They often contain substantial amounts of shortening, oil, or butter to help give them their characteristic soft, cakelike texture.

The breads in this section contain less fat than most quick bread recipes. For this reason, it is especially important not to overbeat the dough. Beating or overmixing develops gluten, one of the proteins in flour, and toughens bread. Good gluten development is desirable in yeast bread, but not in quick breads when you want a tender crumb.

Some of the recipes in this section substitute brown sugar for white sugar, since they aren't high enough in fat to brown naturally. Never overcook these breads, because excess baking will dry them out. Check them at the end of the time specified in the recipe. Muffins and biscuits are done when they are firm on top when you touch them. Recipes for other breads will include how to check for doneness.

Drop Biscuits

———— ◆ ————

My daughter loves these drop biscuits with homemade jam or preserves, just as I loved the higher-fat version when I was young.

They are fast to prepare, because they're mixed in one bowl, dropped into the baking sheet, and cooked only a few minutes. Treat them gently, as there is very little fat to protect them from becoming tough with handling.

If you have leftover biscuits, store them in a plastic bag. When you're ready to serve them, place them on a baking sheet and heat them in a 400°F. oven for two or three minutes.

    2 c. unsifted self-rising flour, or 2 c. all-purpose flour
        plus 1 Tbsp. baking powder and ¼ tsp. salt
    2 Tbsp. tub margarine
    ¼ c. plain nonfat yogurt or fat-free sour cream
    ½ c. plus 2 Tbsp. skim milk

Preheat oven to 450°F., and lightly coat baking sheet with vegetable oil spray.

Put flour and tub margarine in large bowl, and work margarine into flour with your hands or a fork until most of mixture resembles cornmeal in texture. Add yogurt and milk, and mix lightly *just until all flour is moistened*.

Drop dough onto baking sheet by tablespoonfuls. Bake 10 minutes, or until biscuits are lightly browned and cooked through. Serve hot.

YIELD: 14 large biscuits

Each biscuit: 79 calories, 1.8 g fat (20.5% calories from fat), 0.3 g saturated fat, 0.6 g polyunsaturated fat, 0.6 g

monounsaturated fat, 0 mg cholesterol, 13.1 g carbohydrate,
2.2 g protein, 208 mg sodium

EXCHANGES: 1 bread

White Beer Bread

◆

I love making yeast breads, but sometimes I just don't have
enough time. Here's a nice hearty loaf of bread that I can mix
up and bake within an hour.

2½ c. all-purpose flour
4 tsp. baking powder
2 Tbsp. sugar
½ tsp. salt
12 oz. beer, at room temperature

Lightly coat 9-by-5-inch loaf pan with vegetable oil
spray. Preheat oven to 350°F.

Mix together flour, baking powder, sugar, and salt.
Add beer and stir until batter is well mixed. Spoon
batter into baking pan. Set aside at room temperature
about 5 minutes, and then bake 50 minutes, or until
browned on top and cooked throughout.

YIELD: 1 loaf (16 slices)

Each slice: 81 calories, 0.2 g fat (2.2% calories from fat), 0 g
saturated fat, 0 g polyunsaturated fat, 0 g monounsaturated
fat, 0 mg cholesterol, 16.3 g carbohydrate, 1.9 g protein,
126 mg sodium

EXCHANGES: 1 bread

Rye Beer Bread

◆

Rye yeast bread is one of the more difficult breads to make, but rye beer bread is quick and simple as well as delicious.

1½ c. rye flour (Pillsbury or Gold Medal—not stone-
    ground)
1 c. all-purpose or unbleached white flour
2 Tbsp. sugar
1 Tbsp. plus 1 tsp. baking powder
½ tsp. salt
Optional: ½ tsp. caraway seeds
12 oz. beer, at room temperature
¼ c. water

Preheat oven to 350°F. Lightly coat 9-by-5-inch loaf pan with vegetable oil spray.

Mix together rye flour, white flour, sugar, baking powder, salt, and caraway seeds. Add beer and water, and stir until well combined. Spoon batter into loaf pan, and set aside at room temperature 5 minutes. Bake 50 minutes, or until browned on top and cooked through.

Y I E L D : 1 loaf (16 slices)

Each slice: 82 calories, 0.4 g fat (4.4% calories from fat), 0 g saturated fat, <0.1 g polyunsaturated fat, <0.1 g monounsaturated fat, 0 mg cholesterol, 16.3 g carbohydrate, 2.8 g protein, 126 mg sodium

E X C H A N G E S : 1 bread

Irish Soda Bread

———◆———

This recipe makes a rustic, crusty loaf of bread, similar in appearance to a large drop biscuit. The sprinkling of caraway seeds makes it a delicious dinner bread, while the currants add a pleasingly sweet festive touch. Add other dried fruits along with the currants, if you like. Soda bread is easy to make, and it's a wonderful accompaniment to mildly flavored meats such as turkey and baked chicken.

4 c. unsifted unbleached flour
2 Tbsp. sugar
2 tsp. caraway seeds
1 tsp. baking soda
¾ tsp. salt
¾ c. currants or chopped raisins
1¾ c. nonfat buttermilk
1 lightly beaten egg white

Preheat oven to 350°F., and lightly coat baking sheet with vegetable oil spray.

Mix all ingredients except buttermilk and egg white in large bowl until well combined. Add buttermilk, and stir until all flour is moistened. Turn mixture out onto floured work surface, and knead about 10 times, or until dough is in a smooth ball.

Shape dough into a round loaf, place dough on baking sheet, and brush top with egg white. Bake 40 minutes, or until loaf is crusty and lightly browned on top and sounds hollow when lightly thumped. Cover with towel and allow to cool at least 15 minutes before cutting bread into wedges with a serrated knife.

YIELD: 1 loaf (16 servings)

Each serving: 140 calories, 0.4 g fat (2.6% calories from fat), <0.1 g saturated fat, <0.1 g polyunsaturated fat, <0.1 g monounsaturated fat, 0 mg cholesterol, 30 g carbohydrate, 4 g protein, 207 mg sodium

EXCHANGES: 1 bread; 1 fruit

Banana Oatmeal Bread

———◆———

Do you like banana bread but not the half cup or so of oil that most recipes contain? Then here's a recipe without any added fats. It makes a great snack or lunch-box treat.

½ c. boiling water
½ c. oatmeal
¼ c. molasses
¾ c. pureed ripe banana
½ c. sugar
1 large egg
1 tsp. vanilla extract
½ c. plain nonfat yogurt
1 c. flour
1½ tsp. baking powder
½ tsp. baking soda
1 tsp. ground cinnamon
¼ tsp. salt
Optional: ¼ c. pecan pieces

Preheat oven to 350°F. Lightly coat 9-by-5-inch loaf pan with vegetable oil spray.

In large bowl, pour boiling water over oatmeal, stir, cover bowl with plate, and set aside 5 minutes. Then add molasses, bananas, sugar, egg, vanilla extract, and yogurt to oatmeal, and stir until well combined.

In separate bowl, stir together the flour, baking powder, baking soda, cinnamon, and salt until mixture is uniform. Add flour mixture and optional pecans to banana-oatmeal mixture, and stir just until all ingredients are moistened and smooth. Pour batter into loaf pan.

Bake 30–40 minutes, or until bread has browned and begun to pull away from sides of pan. (Top of loaf should not retain a dent when pushed gently with finger.) Cool 5–10 minutes in pan, and then invert loaf onto rack. Serve immediately, or wrap in plastic or aluminum foil and store 1 or 2 days at room temperature or for 1 week or more in refrigerator.

YIELD: 1 loaf (16 slices)

Each slice *without pecans:* 100 calories, 0.7 g fat (6.3% calories from fat), 0.2 g saturated fat, <0.1 g polyunsaturated fat, 0.2 g monounsaturated fat, 17 mg cholesterol, 22 g carbohydrate, 2.1 g protein, 153 mg sodium

EXCHANGES: 1 bread; ½ fruit

Each slice *with pecans:* 124 calories, 3.1 g fat (22.5% calories from fat), 0.4 g saturated fat, 0.7 g polyunsaturated fat, 1.7 g monounsaturated fat, 0 mg cholesterol, 22.4 g carbohydrate, 2.2 g protein, 153 mg sodium

EXCHANGES: 1 bread; ½ fruit; ½ fat

Squash Bread

———◆———

Anyone who's grown squash knows that it's easy to run out of ideas about what to do with it after two or three weeks. Here's a delicious squash bread that can be made with either yellow squash or zucchini. Precooking the squash allows you to puree it and use it in place of oil.

3 c. squash slices
1½ c. all-purpose flour, or 1 c. white and ½ c. whole
    wheat flour
2 tsp. baking powder
½ tsp. baking soda
¼ tsp. salt
2 tsp. ground cinnamon
¼ tsp. ground nutmeg
1 egg
⅔ c. sugar
1 tsp. vanilla extract

Drop squash slices in large pan of boiling water, and simmer for 5–10 minutes, or until tender. Drain squash and mash well by hand, or pulse in food processor until mashed but not thoroughly pureed. Measure out 1½ c. of the squash and set aside to cool. Save any remaining squash for another use.

Preheat oven to 350°F., and lightly coat 8½-by-4½-inch loaf pan with vegetable oil spray.

In one bowl, mix together flour, baking powder, baking soda, salt, cinnamon, and nutmeg. In another, larger bowl, stir together the egg, sugar, vanilla extract, and the 1½ c. squash. When squash mixture is well combined, stir in the dry ingredients, and mix with wooden spoon just until all flour is incorporated.

Pour batter into loaf pan, and bake 30–40 minutes, or until cooked through. Serve hot, or cool to room temperature, wrap with plastic, and store in refrigerator.

YIELD: 1 loaf (10 slices)

Each slice: 125 calories, 0.8 g fat (5.8% calories from fat), 0.2 g saturated fat, 0.1 g polyunsaturated fat, 0.2 g monounsaturated fat, 27 mg cholesterol, 26.9 g carbohydrate, 2.9 g protein, 171 mg sodium

EXCHANGES: 1 bread; 1 vegetable; ½ fruit

Applesauce Waffles

◆

Waffles are so special to my children that they have become our official sleepover breakfast following slumber parties. The children and their friends get as excited about the waffles as about any other part of the event.

Although syrup contains simple sugars and calories, it is fat-free. Other fat-free toppings for waffles are molasses, fruit preserves, and jams.

If your waffle iron makes smaller waffles, this recipe will yield more servings, and each waffle will contain fewer calories and less fat. Be sure to follow the manufacturer's care instructions to keep your waffle iron's finish in good shape.

¾ c. unsweetened applesauce
1 large egg
1 c. skim milk
2 c. unsifted self-rising flour, or 2 c. all-purpose flour, 1
    Tbsp. baking powder, and ¼ tsp. salt

Preheat waffle iron according to manufacturer's instructions. In large bowl, stir together applesauce, egg, and skim milk. When smooth, add flour, and mix only until all flour is moistened. *Do not overmix.*

Lightly coat waffle iron grids with vegetable oil spray. Pour approximately ½ c. batter onto iron for each waffle, depending on size of waffle iron, and bake until medium brown, (1–2 minutes). Repeat for each waffle, being sure to spray grids after each use to prevent sticking. Serve hot.

YIELD: 8 large Belgian waffles

Each waffle: 132 calories, 1.1 g fat (7.5% calories from fat), 0.3 g saturated fat, 0.1 g polyunsaturated fat, 0.3 g monounsaturated fat, 35 mg cholesterol, 25.5 g carbohydrate, 4.5 g protein, 335 mg sodium

EXCHANGES: 1½ bread

Millet Spoon Bread

Despite my Virginia heritage, I've never really liked corn bread. But I love spoon bread.

Here's a low-fat recipe for spoon bread that uses no butter and calls for fewer eggs than the traditional version. This spoon bread also includes millet for a bit more texture.

2 c. cooked millet
½ c. white cornmeal
4 c. skim milk
1 Tbsp. plus 1 tsp. baking powder

½ tsp. salt
2 whole eggs plus 2 egg whites, beaten together

Preheat oven to 325°F., and lightly coat large baking pan with vegetable oil spray. Stir together all ingredients until well mixed, and pour into prepared pan. Bake 50 minutes, or until bread is browned on top and set in the middle. Serve hot.

YIELD: 12 servings

Each serving: 104 calories, 1.2 g fat (10.4% calories from fat), 0.3 g saturated fat, 0.2 g polyunsaturated fat, 0.4 g monounsaturated fat, 46 mg cholesterol, 17.0 g carbohydrate, 5.6 g protein, 272 mg sodium

EXCHANGES: 1 bread; ½ lean meat

MUFFINS

Most muffins contain quite a bit of fat, but the recipes in this section omit all added fats. These muffins are moistened with applesauce or pureed cooked vegetables instead of fats.

These recipes were developed with an eye toward ease of cooking and quick preparation. But if you have the time and wish to work toward an even lighter muffin, you can separate the eggs, add the yolks along with the wet ingredients, beat the egg whites until they're stiff, and fold them into the muffin mixture at the end, just before baking.

Often foods cooked without added fats are lighter in color than those cooked with fats. If you prefer darker muffins, substitute light or dark brown sugar for the white sugar in the recipe.

If you can't find self-rising flour, substitute 1 cup all-purpose flour plus ½ tablespoon baking powder and ⅛ teaspoon salt for each cup of self-rising flour in the recipe.

All of these muffins may be prepared with egg substitutes instead of fresh whole eggs if you'd like to lower fat and cholesterol contents even farther.

Muffins should be eaten hot or stored in a plastic bag after cooling to room temperature. If you plan to keep them more than one day, store them in the refrigerator.

Plain Flour Muffins

◆

These light-textured muffins are somewhat reminiscent of popovers. Enjoy them piping hot from the oven with your favorite jams.

1 egg or equivalent egg substitute
1 c. skim milk
1 c. plus 2 Tbsp. self-rising flour

Preheat oven to 400°F., and lightly coat 6 muffin tins with vegetable oil spray.

Combine egg and skim milk in small bowl. Add flour, and mix just until all flour is moistened. Fill six muffin tins about two-thirds full.

Bake 15–18 minutes, just until cooked through. Muffins will toughen if overcooked. Serve hot.

YIELD: 6 muffins

Each muffin: 94 calories, 1.2 g fat (11.5% calories from fat), 0.3 g saturated fat, 0.1 g polyunsaturated fat, 0.4 g monounsaturated fat, 46 mg cholesterol, 16.2 g carbohydrate, 4.1 g protein, 238 mg sodium

EXCHANGES: 1 bread

Whole Wheat Muffins

———— ◆ ————

1 egg or equivalent egg substitute
2 Tbsp. sugar
⅔ c. skim milk
1 c. whole wheat flour
2 tsp. baking powder
¼ tsp. salt

Preheat oven to 400°F., and lightly coat 8–10 muffin tins with vegetable oil spray.

Mix together egg, sugar, and milk in one bowl, and combine flour, baking powder, and salt in another bowl. Add dry ingredients to milk mixture, and stir just until all flour is incorporated. *Do not overmix*.

Pour batter into muffin tins until tins are almost full. Bake 15–18 minutes, just until cooked through.

Serve hot, or cool muffins to room temperature and store in plastic bag.

YIELD: 8–10 muffins

Each muffin: 71 calories, 0.9 g fat (11.4% calories from fat), 0.2 g saturated fat, <0.1 g polyunsaturated fat, 0.3 g monounsaturated fat, 31 mg cholesterol, 13.2 g carbohydrate, 3.1 g protein, 129 mg sodium

EXCHANGES: 1 bread

Bran Muffins

◆

1 c. unprocessed bran
1 egg or equivalent egg substitute
¼ c. brown sugar or molasses
1 c. skim milk
1 c. self-rising flour

Preheat oven to 400°F., and lightly coat 8–10 muffin tins with vegetable oil spray.

In mixing bowl, combine bran, egg, brown sugar, and skim milk. Set aside for about 5 minutes, and then add flour. Mix only until all flour is incorporated.

Pour batter into muffin tins, filling each about three-quarters full. Bake 15–18 minutes, or until cooked through. Serve immediately, or cool thoroughly and store in plastic bag.

YIELD: 8–10 muffins

Each muffin: 87 calories, 0.8 g fat (8.3% calories from fat), 0.2 g saturated fat, <0.1 g polyunsaturated fat, 0.3 g monounsaturated fat, 31 mg cholesterol, 17.0 g carbohydrate, 2.8 g protein, 161 mg sodium

EXCHANGES: 1 bread

Multigrain Muffins

◆

This is a fun recipe that yields an interesting muffin for grain lovers.

¼ c. oatmeal
¼ c. cornmeal
¼ c. whole wheat *or* rye flour
¼ c. bulgur wheat
¼ c. whole wheat couscous
¼ c. unprocessed wheat bran
1 shredded wheat cake, finely crumbled
½ tsp. salt
½ c. raisins
¼–½ c. molasses
2 c. boiling water
1 whole egg plus 2 egg whites
½ c. unsweetened applesauce
½ c. plain nonfat yogurt or sour cream
Optional: ¼ c. pecan pieces
4 tsp. baking powder
2 c. unbleached or all-purpose flour

Preheat oven to 400°F., and lightly coat 20 muffin tins with vegetable oil spray.

In large bowl, mix first ten ingredients together. Pour the boiling water over them, and stir until well mixed. Cover bowl, and set aside for 1 hour at room temperature or up to 2 days in refrigerator.

With wooden spoon, stir eggs, applesauce, yogurt, and optional pecans into batter. Combine the baking powder and the unbleached or all-purpose flour, add to batter, and stir just until flour is well incorporated.

Fill tins with batter, and bake 20 minutes, or until browned and cooked through. Best when served hot.

YIELD: About 20 muffins

Each muffin without pecans: 106 calories, 0.6 g fat (5.1% calories from fat), 0.1 g saturated fat, <0.1 g polyunsaturated fat, 0.1 g monounsaturated fat, 14 mg cholesterol, 22.0 g carbohydrate, 3.2 g protein, 131 mg sodium

EXCHANGES: 1½ breads

Each muffin with pecans: 125 calories, 2.7 g fat (19.4% calories from fat)

EXCHANGES: 1½ breads; ½ fat

Apple Muffins

◆

¾ c. unsweetened applesauce
1 egg or equivalent egg substitute
¼ c. sugar
½ tsp. vanilla extract
1 tsp. ground cinnamon
¼ tsp. ground nutmeg
1¼ c. self-rising flour
¾ c. diced apples

Preheat oven to 400°F., and lightly coat 8–10 muffin tins with vegetable oil spray.

Mix together applesauce, egg, sugar, and vanilla extract in one bowl, and combine cinnamon, nutmeg, and flour in another bowl. Add dry ingredients to wet ingredients, and mix only until all flour is incorporated. Fold in apples. Pour batter into muffin tins, filling almost full. Bake 15–18 minutes, or just until cooked through. Serve hot, or store in plastic bag when thoroughly cooled.

YIELD: 8–10 muffins

Each muffin: 103 calories, 0.8 g fat (7.0% calories from fat), 0.2 g saturated fat, 0.1 g polyunsaturated fat, 0.3 g monounsaturated fat, 30 mg cholesterol, 21.8 g carbohydrate, 2.2 g protein, 180 mg sodium

EXCHANGES: 1 bread; ½ fruit

Poppy Seed–Lemon Muffins

◆

Don't eat these muffins before taking a drug test. There have been reports of poppy seeds causing false positive results for opiates!

> ¾ c. unsweetened applesauce
> 1 egg or equivalent egg substitute
> ½ tsp. vanilla extract
> ½ c. sugar
> Juice and zest of one medium lemon
> 2 Tbsp. poppy seeds
> 1¼ c. self-rising flour

Preheat oven to 400°F., and lightly coat 8–10 muffin tins with vegetable oil spray.

Stir together applesauce, egg, vanilla extract, sugar, lemon juice and zest, and poppy seeds. Add flour, and stir just until flour is well incorporated.

Pour batter into muffin tins, filling each almost full. Bake 15–18 minutes, or until cooked through. Serve hot, or cool muffins to room temperature and store in plastic bag.

Y I E L D : 8–10 muffins

Each muffin: 113 calories, 0.8 g fat (6.4% calories from fat), 0.2 g saturated fat, <0.1 g polyunsaturated fat, 0.2 g monounsaturated fat, 30 mg cholesterol, 24.5 g carbohydrate, 2.2 g protein, 180 mg sodium

E X C H A N G E S : 1 bread; 1 fruit

Orange Muffins

◆

¾ c. unsweetened applesauce
1 egg or equivalent egg substitute
½ tsp. vanilla extract
½ c. sugar
Juice and zest of one-half small juice orange
1¼ c. self-rising flour

Preheat oven to 400°F., and lightly coat 8–10 muffin tins with vegetable oil spray.

Mix together applesauce, egg, vanilla extract, sugar, and orange juice and zest. Add flour, and stir just until flour is thoroughly incorporated. Pour batter into muffin tins, filling each almost full. Bake 14–18 minutes, just until cooked through. Do not overcook, or muffins will be tough.

Serve immediately, or cool muffins to room temperature and store in plastic bag.

YIELD: 8–10 muffins

Each muffin: 114 calories, 0.8 g fat (6.3% calories from fat), 0.2 g saturated fat, <0.1 g polyunsaturated fat, 0.2 g monounsaturated fat, 30 mg cholesterol, 24.6 g carbohydrate, 2.2 g protein, 180 mg sodium

EXCHANGES: 1 bread; ½ fruit

Blueberry Muffins

◆

¾ c. unsweetened applesauce
1 egg or equivalent egg substitute
½ tsp. vanilla extract
½ c. light brown sugar
1¼ c. self-rising flour
¾ c. frozen or canned blueberries, well drained

Preheat oven to 400°F., and lightly coat 8–10 muffin tins with vegetable oil spray.

Combine applesauce, egg, vanilla extract, and sugar in large bowl. Add flour, and mix until flour is almost all incorporated. Fold in blueberries until they are well distributed throughout batter. Do not overmix, or batter will be blue.

Pour batter into muffin tins, filling each almost full. Bake 15–18 minutes, or just until cooked through. Do not overcook, or muffins will be tough.

Serve immediately, or cool muffins to room temperature and store in plastic bag.

YIELD: 8–10 muffins

Each muffin: 123 calories, 0.9 g fat (6.6% calories from fat), 0.2 g saturated fat, <0.1 g polyunsaturated fat, 0.2 g monounsaturated fat, 30 mg cholesterol, 26.8 g carbohydrate, 2.2 g protein, 181 mg sodium

EXCHANGES: 1 bread; 1 fruit

Carrot-Raisin Muffins
◆

¾ c. unsweetened applesauce
1 egg or equivalent egg substitute
½ tsp. vanilla extract
¼ c. sugar
1¼ c. self-rising flour
1 tsp. ground cinnamon
¾ c. grated carrots
¼ c. raisins

Preheat oven to 400°F., and lightly coat 8–10 muffin tins with vegetable oil spray.

Combine applesauce, egg, vanilla extract, and sugar in large bowl, and mix well. Add flour and cinnamon, and stir until flour is almost all incorporated. Stir in carrots and raisins until they are evenly distributed. Pour batter into tins, filling them almost full. Bake 15–18 minutes, or until cooked through. Do not overcook, or muffins will be tough.

YIELD: 8–10 muffins

Each muffin: 112 calories, 0.8 g fat (6.4% calories from fat), 0.2 g saturated fat, 0.1 g polyunsaturated fat, 0.2 g

monounsaturated fat, 30 mg cholesterol, 24.2 g carbohydrate, 2.4 g protein, 184 mg sodium

EXCHANGES: 1 bread; ½ fruit

Squash Muffins

◆

Follow recipe for Squash Bread (page 200), but cook in muffin tins lightly coated with vegetable oil spray. Bake 15–18 minutes, or until cooked through.

YIELD: 10 muffins

Each muffin: 125 calories, 0.8 g fat (5.8% calories from fat), 0.2 g saturated fat, 0.1 g polyunsaturated fat, 0.2 g monounsaturated fat, 27 mg cholesterol, 26.9 g carbohydrate, 2.9 g protein, 171 mg sodium

EXCHANGES: 1 bread; 1 vegetable; ½ fruit

Hearty Oatmeal Spice Muffins

◆

These oatmeal muffins are hearty and chewy—full of the goodness of oatmeal. You can omit the molasses, if you wish, and increase the sugar to ½ cup.

    1 c. uncooked oatmeal
    1 tsp. ground cinnamon
    ¼ tsp. ground nutmeg
    ¼ tsp. ground ginger
    ¼ c. sugar
    ¼ c. molasses

1 egg or equivalent egg substitute
1 tsp. vanilla extract
1 c. skim milk
1 c. self-rising flour

Preheat oven to 400°F., and lightly coat 8–10 muffin tins with vegetable oil spray.

Stir together all ingredients except flour, and set mixture aside for 5–10 minutes. Add flour, and stir just until thoroughly incorporated. Pour batter into muffin tins, filling almost full. Bake 14–18 minutes, just until cooked through. Serve hot, or cool muffins to room temperature and store in plastic bag.

YIELD: 8–10 muffins

Each muffin: 131 calories. 1.5 g fat (10.3% calories from fat), 0.4 g saturated fat, <0.1 g polyunsaturated fat, 0.3 g monounsaturated fat, 31 mg cholesterol, 24.8 g carbohydrate, 4.4 g protein, 194 mg sodium

EXCHANGES: 1½ breads

Banana-Oatmeal Muffins

———◆———

1 c. uncooked oatmeal
¼ c. sugar
1 c. well-mashed or pureed overripe bananas
½ c. skim milk
1 egg or equivalent egg substitute
1 tsp. vanilla extract
¼ c. brown sugar
1 c. plus 2 Tbsp. self-rising flour

Preheat oven to 400°F., and lightly coat 8–10 muffin tins with vegetable oil spray.

Stir together all ingredients except flour, and set mixture aside for 5–10 minutes. Add flour, and stir just until thoroughly incorporated. Pour batter into muffin tins, filling almost full. Bake 14–18 minutes, just until cooked through. Serve hot, or cool muffins to room temperature and store in plastic bag.

YIELD: 8–10 muffins

Each muffin: 139 calories, 1.6 g fat (10.4% calories from fat), 0.4 g saturated fat, <0.1 g polyunsaturated fat, 0.3 g monounsaturated fat, 31 mg cholesterol, 28.1 g carbohydrate, 3.9 g protein, 155 mg sodium

EXCHANGES: 1 bread; 1 fruit

Corn Muffins

When buying a cornmeal mix, be sure that it says "self-rising" on the package. The ingredient list should include flour.

    1 c. creamed corn
    ½ Tbsp. sugar
    1 large egg
    ¼ c. skim milk
    2 Tbsp. chopped onion
    1 c. self-rising cornmeal mix

Preheat oven to 400°F., and lightly coat 8–10 muffin tins with vegetable oil spray. Mix together all ingredients until cornmeal is completely moistened. Pour batter into muffin tins until almost full. Bake 14–16 minutes, or until cooked through.

YIELD: 8–10 muffins

Each muffin: 82 calories, 1.2 g fat (13.2% calories from fat), 0.2 g saturated fat, <0.1 g polyunsaturated fat, 0.3 g monounsaturated fat, 31 mg cholesterol, 16.0 g carbohydrate, 2.6 g protein, 230 mg sodium

EXCHÁNGES: 1 bread

Southwestern Corn Muffins

◆

These muffins, with their unusual flavor combination, are fun to serve with Mexican or southwestern meals.

½ c. creamed corn
½ c. hot or mild salsa
1 large egg
¼ c. skim milk
1 c. self-rising cornmeal mix

Preheat over to 400°F., and lightly coat 8–10 muffin tins with vegetable oil spray. Mix together all ingredients until cornmeal is thoroughly moistened. Pour batter into muffin tins until almost full, and bake 14–16 minutes, until muffins are cooked through.

YIELD: 8–10 muffins

Each muffin: 75 calories, 1.1 g fat (13.1% calories from fat), 0.2 g saturated fat, <0.1 g polyunsaturated fat, 0.3 g

monounsaturated fat, 31 mg cholesterol, 14.3 g carbohydrate, 2.5 g protein, 277 mg sodium

EXCHANGES: 1 bread

Ginger Muffins with Lemon Sauce

——◆——

The spicy aroma of ginger and cinnamon will fill your house when you bake these muffins. Top them with the Lemon Sauce and eat them with a fork for a special treat, or serve them plain, if you wish. Either way, make enough for everyone to have seconds!

1 c. whole wheat flour
⅔ c. all-purpose or unbleached flour
¼ c. sugar
1½ tsp. baking soda
1 tsp. ground ginger
¾ tsp. ground cinnamon
½ tsp. salt
½ c. boiling water
¾ c. molasses
¾ c. unsweetened applesauce
1 egg or equivalent egg substitute
Optional: 1 tsp. lemon zest

Lemon Sauce:
Zest of 1 lemon
½ c. sugar
2–3 Tbsp. fresh lemon juice
1 Tbsp. cornstarch mixed with ½ c. water

Preheat oven to 350°F., and lightly coat 18 muffin tins with vegetable oil spray.

Whisk together whole wheat flour, all-purpose flour, sugar, baking soda, ginger, cinnamon, and salt until no lumps remain. In separate bowl, pour boiling water into molasses, and stir. Add applesauce, egg, and, if desired, lemon zest. Add molasses mixture to dry ingredients, and stir only until all flour is incorporated and mixture is relatively free of lumps.

Spoon batter into muffin tins, filling about two-thirds full, and bake 15 minutes, until muffins are cooked through.

At serving time, combine all Lemon Sauce ingredients in small saucepan. Cook, stirring constantly, until sauce boils and thickens. Remove from heat. Serve over hot Ginger Muffins.

YIELD: **Approx. 18 muffins**

Each muffin with 2 Tbsp. lemon sauce: 122 calories, 0.5 g fat (3.7% calories from fat), <0.1 g saturated fat, <0.1 g polyunsaturated fat, 0.1 g monounsaturated fat, 15 mg cholesterol, 28.7 carbohydrate, 1.7 g protein, 169 mg sodium

EXCHANGES: **1 bread; 1 fruit**

Pumpkin Muffins

◆

2 c. unsifted all-purpose flour
1 Tbsp. baking powder
1 tsp. baking soda
2 tsp. ground cinnamon
½ tsp. ground nutmeg
½ tsp. ground allspice
¼ tsp. ground mace
1 tsp. salt
2 c. sugar
1 tsp. vanilla extract
2 large eggs
1 can (16 oz.) pumpkin puree

Preheat oven to 350°F., and lightly coat 18 muffin tins with vegetable oil spray.

In small mixing bowl, stir together flour, baking powder, baking soda, spices, and salt. Set aside. In large mixing bowl, use wire whisk to combine sugar, vanilla extract, eggs, and pumpkin until very smooth. Fold in dry ingredients, and mix only until all white flour disappears. Spoon batter into prepared muffin tins, filling about two-thirds full, and bake 15–18 minutes, or until muffins are thoroughly cooked.

YIELD: Approx. 18 muffins

Each muffin: 150 calories, 0.8 g fat (4.8% calories from fat), 0.2 g saturated fat, <0.1 g polyunsaturated fat, 0.3 g monounsaturated fat, 30 mg cholesterol, 34.2 g carbohydrate, 2.4 g protein, 236 mg sodium

EXCHANGES: 1 bread, 2 fruits

DESSERTS

———◆———

Ask people who have cut back on their fat intake what foods they miss the most in their new eating style, and you'll most likely hear them mourning the loss of their favorite desserts. There's no doubt that many people *love* desserts and that most of the traditional ones are loaded with fat and calories.

Here is a whole section of enjoyable low-fat desserts, many of which are already favorites of *The Low-Fat Epicure* subscribers. While the main emphasis has been on eliminating added fats such as oil, margarine, butter, and shortening, some of these desserts have also seen reductions in sugar and the use of whole wheat flour in place of white flour when the quality of the product isn't noticeably reduced.

Please note that exchange information is included with all of these recipes, just as with the other recipes throughout the book. I hope this information will be helpful, especially for people on calorie-restricted meal plans that use exchange lists. You may notice "fruit exchanges" listed at times when fruit isn't in the dessert; this is probably because the food contains sugar. Since sugar contains only carbohydrate and no protein or fat, it fits best into the fruit exchange. Remember, however, that these simple sugars, unlike fruits, contain no nutrients other than calories. Foods containing significant amounts of simple sugars, such as table sugar, fructose, honey, molasses, and corn syrup, should be used as special-occasion foods.

It is important for diabetics to realize that the inclusion of exchange information in this section does not automatically mean that these foods are suitable for diabetics. Only you and your physician can decide whether sugar is suitable for your individual diet.

CAKES

Moist Chocolate Cake

———◆———

You shouldn't feel guilty when enjoying this chocolate cake with frosting. This cake gets its intense chocolate flavor and dark color from Hershey's European-style cocoa powder—the kind that comes in a silver tin—although any alkali-processed cocoa will do.

1 c. Hershey's European-style or any alkali-processed
   cocoa powder
2¼ c. cake flour
2 c. sugar
1 tsp. baking powder
1 tsp. baking soda
½ tsp. salt
2 eggs
1½ c. water
2 tsp. vanilla extract
2 Tbsp. vegetable oil

Preheat oven to 350°F., and lightly coat two 10-inch round cake pans with vegetable oil spray.

In large bowl, combine cocoa powder, cake flour, sugar, baking powder, baking soda, and salt, and stir together with wire whisk or spoon until mixture is light and uniform and no lumps remain. In smaller bowl, mix together the eggs, water, vanilla extract, and oil until smooth.

Add egg mixture to dry ingredients. Mix with wooden spoon just until batter is smooth and creamy. Pour batter into prepared cake pans, dividing it evenly between the two. Bake on middle rack of oven 20–25 minutes, until no longer wet when pressed lightly in middle of pan.

Remove from oven, cool in pans 10 minutes, and then turn out onto rack. If desired, frost when completely cooled (frosting recipe follows).

YIELD: 16 wedges

Each serving (¹⁄₁₆ of cake), without frosting: 193 calories, 3.3 g total fat (15.1% calories from fat), 0.5 g saturated fat, 1.1 g polyunsaturated fat, 0.7 g monounsaturated fat, 38 mg cholesterol, 38 g carbohydrate, 3 g protein, 171 mg sodium

EXCHANGES: 1 bread; 1½ fruits; ½ fat

VARIATION: For 16 Chocolate Cupcakes, use one-half recipe, and frost with one-half frosting recipe. Nutritional content for each cupcake is one-half that of one serving of cake plus one-half that of one serving of frosting.

Chocolate Frosting

◆

This recipe uses light cream cheese to give it the perfect consistency for frosting a layer cake.

½ c. cocoa powder
4 c. confectioners' sugar
⅛ tsp. salt
4 oz. light cream cheese
3 Tbsp plus up to 3 tsp. skim milk
1 tsp. vanilla extract

In large mixing bowl, stir together the cocoa powder, 1 c. of the confectioners' sugar, and the salt. Add the light cream cheese, and use electric mixer—with whisk beater, if available—to beat the mixture until creamy. Add the 3 Tbsp. skim milk and the vanilla extract, and beat again until creamy. Add rest of confectioners' sugar, beating until thick and smooth. If necessary, add rest of skim milk, 1 teaspoon at a time, until frosting is of good spreading consistency.

YIELD: Enough to frost one 2-layer cake (16 servings)

Each serving: 124 calories, 1.6 g fat (11.5% calories from fat), 0.8 g saturated fat, 0 g polyunsaturated fat, 0 g monounsaturated fat, 3 mg cholesterol, 27 g carbohydrate, 2 g protein, 59 mg sodium

EXCHANGES: 1 bread; 1 fruit

Carrot Cake with Sour Cream Topping
———◆———

This recipe makes a very moist carrot cake. I like it best made with fresh pureed carrots (cook and puree enough for two cakes at once), but for days when you're really rushed, I've also included directions for using baby food carrots.

  2 c. all-purpose flour (plus 2 Tbsp. if using baby food
     carrots)
  1 Tbsp. plus 1 tsp. baking powder
  ½ tsp. salt
  2 tsp. ground cinnamon
  2 c. pureed carrots (directions follow), or 3 jars (6 oz.
     each) baby food carrots

2 eggs
2 c. sugar
½ c. raisins
1 c. shredded carrots

Topping (optional):
1 c. fat-free sour cream or plain nonfat yogurt
¼ c. sugar, or more to taste

Preheat oven to 350°F., and lightly coat bundt or tube pan with vegetable oil spray.

In small bowl, stir together flour, baking powder, salt, and cinnamon. In larger bowl, combine carrot puree, eggs, and sugar until mixture is very smooth. Add flour mixture, and stir with wooden spoon (do *not* use mixer) *just* until all flour is incorporated. Add raisins and shredded carrots, and stir until they are evenly distributed.

Pour batter into prepared pan, and bake 40–50 minutes, just until cooked through. (When you press top of cake gently, it should feel firm and you shouldn't leave finger marks.)

Cool in pan 5–10 minutes, and then invert onto rack. Serve warm, or cool cake to room temperature and store in airtight container. If you desire sour cream topping, mix together the sour cream and sugar, and refrigerate in separate container until ready to use. Spoon a dollop of topping onto each serving.

YIELD: 1 cake (16 servings)

Each serving (without topping): 201 calories, 1.0 g fat (4.4% calories from fat), 0.2 g saturated fat, 0.1 g polyunsaturated fat, 0.3 g monounsaturated fat, 35 mg cholesterol, 45.3 g carbohydrate, 4.0 g protein, 160 mg sodium

Each tablespoon of topping: approx. 30 calories, 0 g fat (0% calories from fat)

E X C H A N G E S : **1 bread; 1 vegetable; 1½ fruit**

VARIATION: To make your own Carrot Puree: Scrub 1 pound of carrots well. (If you clean them well enough, there is no need to peel them.) Grate 1 cup of the carrots and set aside to use in the cake recipe. Cut the rest up coarsely, discarding stem ends, and place in saucepan. Add water to half the depth of the carrots, cover, and cook until tender. Drain water, reserving some of it, and place carrots in food processor or food mill. Puree the carrots, returning just enough of the liquid to yield a thick, smooth puree.

Pumpkin Cake with Almond Glaze

◆

Our Christmas dessert table always had pumpkin pie on it. This moist, spicy cake reminds me of that custardy pie, but it omits the high-fat crust. When baked in a pretty mold and glazed as directed, this cake becomes a showpiece, even for the inexperienced cook. It's delicious topped with a dollop of Lite Cool Whip at less than one gram of fat per tablespoon.

Do not beat this cake with an electric mixer, as that would develop the flour's gluten and toughen the cake. Treat this like muffin batter, gently folding the dry ingredients in at the end only until the white flour mixture disappears.

2 c. unsifted cake flour
1 Tbsp. baking powder
1 tsp baking soda
2 tsp. ground cinnamon

½ tsp. ground nutmeg
½ tsp. ground allspice
¼ tsp. ground mace
1 tsp. salt
2 c. sugar
1 tsp. vanilla extract
2 large eggs
1 can (16 oz.) pumpkin puree

Glaze:
½ c. confectioners' sugar
1 shake *each* of ground cinnamon, nutmeg, allspice,
    and mace
1 Tbsp. orange juice concentrate
1 tsp. water
1 Tbsp. sliced almonds

Preheat oven to 350°F., and lightly coat bundt or tube pan with vegetable oil spray.

In small mixing bowl, stir together the flour, baking powder, baking soda, spices, and salt. Set aside. In a large mixing bowl, combine sugar, vanilla extract, eggs, and pumpkin, whisking until mixture is very smooth. Gently stir in dry ingredients, and mix only until all the white flour disappears.

Pour cake batter into prepared pan, and bake 30–40 minutes, or until cake is no longer wet on top and is lightly browned. Cool in pan 10 minutes, and then invert onto rack.

To prepare glaze, mix confectioners' sugar, spices, orange juice concentrate, and water together until they form a very smooth paste. Heat on stovetop or in the microwave oven just until barely pourable. Place cooled cake on cake dish, pour glaze over cake, and sprinkle almond slices evenly over top. Serve immediately, or wait until glaze hardens to cover with plastic wrap until ready to serve.

Y I E L D : 1 cake (16 servings)

Each serving (¹⁄₁₆ of cake): 180 calories, 1.4 g fat (7% calories from fat), 0.3 g saturated fat, 0.2 g polyunsaturated fat, 0.6 g monounsaturated fat, 34 mg cholesterol, 41.0 g carbohydrate, 2.2 g protein, 256 mg sodium

E X C H A N G E S : 1 bread; 2 fruits

Sweet Potato Round Cakes

———◆———

Wrap these cakes in plastic wrap and tie them with pretty ribbons to make inexpensive gifts for teachers, neighbors, and friends.

    2 clean 16-oz. metal cans
    1¼ c. all-purpose flour
    1 tsp. ground cinnamon
    ½ tsp. ground nutmeg
    ½ tsp. baking soda
    ¼ tsp. salt
    1 can (16 oz.) sweet potatoes packed in light syrup,
        drained
    ½ c. sugar
    ¼ c. molasses
    1 egg
    ½ c. raisins

Preheat oven to 350°F., and lightly coat inside of cans with vegetable oil spray. In large bowl, mix together flour, cinnamon, nutmeg, baking soda, and salt until well combined.

Place drained sweet potatoes in bowl of food processor, and process until smooth. Remove from bowl. Measure out 1¼ c. pureed sweet potatoes, and return to food processor with sugar, molasses, and egg. Process until very smooth. (Reserve unused sweet potatoes for another use.)

Add potato mixture to dry ingredients, and stir just until all flour is absorbed. Fold in raisins. *Do not overmix*. Spoon batter into cans. Bake 50–60 minutes, or until cakes are firm to the touch or cake tester comes out clean. Cool in cans 15 minutes before transferring to rack.

YIELD: 12 servings

Each serving: 135 calories, 0.6 g fat (4.0% calories from fat), 0.1 g saturated fat, <0.1 g polyunsaturated fat, 0.2 g monounsaturated fat, 23 mg cholesterol, 30.9 g carbohydrate, 2.2 g protein, 106 mg sodium

EXCHANGES: 1 bread; 1 fruit

Cranberry-Apple Cake

———— ◆ ————

Here's a moist, delicious holiday cake without any oil, margarine, butter, or shortening. Be sure to freeze several bags of fresh cranberries when they are in season so that you can make this dessert all year round. You can also use dried cranberries, which are becoming more widely available; soak them in hot water until plump before mixing your batter.

1½ c. cranberries
2¼ c. cake flour
1½ c. sugar
1 Tbsp. baking powder
½ tsp. baking soda
2 tsp. ground cinnamon
½ tsp. salt
1¼ c. unsweetened applesauce
2 eggs
½ c. skim milk
1 tsp. vanilla extract
¼ c. toasted pecans, in small pieces
1 tsp. (approx.) confectioners' sugar

Preheat oven to 350°F., and lightly coat bundt pan with vegetable oil spray. Grind cranberries coarsely (some should remain almost whole), and set aside.

Combine flour, sugar, baking powder, baking soda, cinnamon, and salt in medium bowl. Whisk together until all ingredients are well distributed. In larger bowl, stir together applesauce, eggs, skim milk, and vanilla extract until well combined. Add dry ingredients, and stir with wooden spoon just until all flour is mixed in and batter is smooth. Fold in cranberries and pecans, and pour into prepared bundt pan. Smooth top, and place in center of oven.

Bake 40–50 minutes, or until surface is golden brown, cake pulls slightly away from sides of pan, and cake feels firm when surface is gently pushed. Remove from oven, cool in pan 10 minutes, and then invert onto rack and leave until fully cooled. (Cake will be slightly wet inside until completely cooled.) Store tightly covered. Sprinkle with confectioners' sugar before slicing.

YIELD: 16 servings

Each serving (¹⁄₁₆ of cake): 171 calories, 3.3 g fat (17.3% calories from fat), 0.4 g saturated fat, 0.7 g polyunsaturated fat, 1.8 g monounsaturated fat, 34 mg cholesterol, 34 g carbohydrate, 2.4 g protein, 123 mg sodium

EXCHANGES: 1 bread; 1 fruit; ½ fat

Gingerbread with Lemon Sauce

◆

If my grandmother, Mrs. Irma Lyell, were still alive, she would heartily approve of this gingerbread. This recipe is the closest I've ever come to hers—and it can be made practically fat-free if you use an egg substitute instead of an egg. The whole wheat flour adds extra fiber.

    1 c. whole wheat flour
    ⅔ c. bleached or unbleached all-purpose flour
    ½ c. sugar
    1½ tsp. baking soda
    1 tsp. ground ginger

¾ tsp. ground cinnamon
½ tsp. salt
½ c. boiling water
¾ c. molasses
¾ c. unsweetened applesauce
1 egg or equivalent egg substitute

Lemon Sauce:
Zest of one lemon
½ c. sugar
2–3 Tbsp. fresh lemon juice
1 Tbsp. cornstarch mixed with ½ c. water

Preheat oven to 350°F., and lightly coat 8-inch-square baking pan with vegetable oil spray. Whisk together whole wheat flour, all-purpose flour, sugar, baking soda, ginger, cinnamon, and salt until no lumps remain. In a separate bowl, pour boiling water into the molasses, and stir. Add applesauce and egg, and combine well. Add molasses mixture to dry ingredients, and stir only until all flour is mixed in and mixture is relatively free of lumps. Pour mixture into prepared pan, and bake 35–40 minutes, until cooked in center. Remove from oven to cooling rack. After 30 minutes, wrap pan tightly until ready to serve.

Mix all Lemon Sauce ingredients in small saucepan. Cook, stirring constantly, until sauce boils and thickens. Remove from heat. Serve warm or cool over gingerbread squares.

Y I E L D : **12 servings**

Each serving (¹⁄₁₂ of gingerbread and 2 Tbsp. sauce): 185 calories, 0.7 g fat (3.4% calories from fat), 0.1 g saturated

fat, <0.1 g polyunsaturated fat, 0.2 g monounsaturated fat, 23 mg cholesterol, 43.5 g carbohydrate, 2.6 g protein, 256 mg sodium

EXCHANGES: 1 bread; 2 fruits

Angel Food Cake

◆

In cooking classes I've taught, people have enjoyed seeing me make angel food cake. It really is not difficult. If you follow the instructions carefully, you should have no trouble making a delicious cake. It's wonderful served with fresh berries on top.

    1 c. cake flour
    ¼ c. plus ¾ c. sugar
    10 egg whites
    ½ tsp. salt
    1 tsp. cream of tartar
    1 tsp. vanilla extract

Stir together the flour and the ¼ c. sugar, and then sift mixture or shake it through a sieve. Set aside. In separate bowl, beat egg whites on medium speed until frothy. Add salt and cream of tartar. Continue beating on highest speed until whites reach the soft peak stage (when you lift mixer, egg whites peak but then fall softly). Continue to beat, adding the remaining ¾ c. sugar slowly, until egg whites are glossy and just start to hold a peak firmly when mixer is lifted. (Do not overbeat.) Add vanilla extract, and beat just long enough to mix.

Preheat oven to 350°F.

Sift flour mixture over egg whites, a little at a time, and fold flour into whites with spatula, taking care to go slowly and gently so that egg whites will keep their volume.

When flour is all incorporated, spoon batter into *ungreased* tube pan. Run a knife through the batter to remove any air pockets, and then smooth the surface. Bake 50 minutes, or until cake is lightly browned on top and springs back when pressed in the middle.

Remove from oven, and invert pan on a towel to allow steam to escape so bottom of cake will not get soggy. When completely cool, run a knife around inner edges of pan to loosen cake, and remove it from pan.

YIELD: 12 servings

Each serving (¹⁄₁₂ of cake): 107 calories, 0 g fat (0% calories from fat), 0 g saturated fat, 0 g polyunsaturated fat, 0 g monounsaturated fat, 0 mg cholesterol, 23.4 g carbohydrate, 3.4 g protein, 131 mg sodium

EXCHANGES: 1½ breads

Chocolate Angel Food Cake

◆

This is a real lunch-box treat in our family. It also makes a decadent dessert when topped with vanilla frozen yogurt and Hershey's chocolate syrup, which is very low in fat. It has twice the cocoa powder of many chocolate angel food cakes, so it satisfies even my husband's "chocolate tooth."

½ c. cocoa powder
½ c. all-purpose flour
¼ c. plus 1 c. sugar
10 large egg whites
¼ tsp. salt
1 tsp. cream of tartar
1 tsp. vanilla

Preheat oven to 350°F. In medium bowl, mix together cocoa powder, flour, and the ¼ c. sugar. Sift mixture or shake it through a sieve two or three times, until the mixture is fine and uniform. Set aside.

Beat egg whites until frothy. Add salt and cream of tartar and continue beating until whites turn from yellow to a soft white mass. Add the remaining 1 c. sugar slowly, one or two tablespoons at a time, while beating, and continue beating until whites just begin to hold a firm peak.

With spatula, gently fold flour mixture into egg whites, a little bit at a time, taking care not to deflate the egg whites. When batter is uniform, pour into *ungreased* tube pan, and bake 45–50 minutes, or until cooked through.

YIELD: 12 servings

Each serving (1/12 of cake): 127 calories, 0.6 g fat (4.2% calories from fat), 0 g saturated fat, 0 g polyunsaturated fat, 0 g monounsaturated fat, 0 mg cholesterol, 26.5 g carbohydrate, 4.2 g protein, 88 mg sodium

EXCHANGES: 2 breads

Cocoa Angel Roll

———◆———

I never succeeded at a cake roll until I came up with this recipe. The angel food base is perfect, as it is not as tender and breakable as cakes containing fat. You'll be proud of how accomplished you'll feel and look when you serve this!

1½ quarts fat-free or low-fat frozen dessert (light ice
    cream or frozen yogurt)
¾ c. cake flour
½ c. cocoa powder
½ c. plus ½ c. sugar
9 egg whites
1 tsp. cream of tartar
1 tsp. vanilla extract
Optional: Hershey's chocolate syrup

Remove frozen dessert from freezer, and set aside at room temperature. Preheat oven to 350°F. Line bottom of ungreased 17-by-11-inch baking sheet with ungreased parchment, and set aside.

Stir flour, cocoa powder, and ½ c. of the sugar together in a small bowl, and set aside. In separate bowl, beat egg whites until foamy, and add cream of tartar. Beat in remaining ½ c. sugar, a tablespoon at a time, until egg whites just start to hold a stiff peak. Do not beat past this point. Stir in vanilla extract.

Pour flour-cocoa mixture into egg whites, and fold it in gently until flour is incorporated. Pour batter into parchment-lined baking sheet, and level with spatula. Bake 15 minutes, or *just* until cooked through. Watch carefully after 10 minutes, and do not overcook.

Remove cake from oven. After 1 minute, invert onto large towel. Immediately roll cake up slowly, starting along one of the long edges, leaving the towel in the roll and using it to guide the cake into the roll. Set rolled-up cake aside 4–5 minutes while you get frozen dessert ready to spread. If frozen dessert is not yet soft enough to spread, microwave it for a few seconds or dip container in warm water.

Unroll cake, and remove towel. Quickly spread frozen dessert over entire surface of cake up to 1 inch from all edges. Carefully roll cake back up, taking care not to let it split. Place roll on baking sheet, seam down. Cover well with plastic wrap, and place in freezer immediately. Freeze until firm.

Remove from freezer 5–10 minutes before serving. Cut into 1-inch-thick slices, place on plates, and, if desired, drizzle small amount chocolate syrup on top.

YIELD: 16 servings

Each serving (without syrup): 154 calories, 2.5 g fat (14.6% calories from fat), 1.3 g saturated fat, <0.1 g polyunsaturated fat, 0.6 g monounsaturated fat, 7 mg cholesterol, 28.4 g carbohydrate, 4.8 g protein, 69 mg sodium

EXCHANGES: 1 bread; ½ milk; ½ fruit; ½ fat

Ice Cream Cake

◆

The first time I made this cake with my children, we had a wonderful time. Before making the angel food cake, we all read together *The High Rise Glorious Skittle Skat Roarious Sky Pie Angel Food Cake* by Nancy Willard, and then we pretended that the angels appeared to give our cake special powers, too. We even put a thimble in the cake before baking it, so that whoever got the slice with the thimble would have extra special luck all year round.

This can be a fun cake for the Fourth of July. Decorate your cake with vanilla frozen yogurt or ice milk and top with blueberries and strawberries or red raspberries. If you can find small American flags, place them in a circle around the top.

Use a store-bought cake for this treat, if you wish, or make one from scratch, using the recipe on page 234.

½ gallon fat-free or low-fat frozen yogurt or ice milk
1 angel food cake
Optional: Berries and flags for topping

Leave the yogurt or ice milk at room temperature for 30 minutes, or until softened just enough to spread, but don't let it melt.

Slice cake horizontally to make two or three layers. Spread softened frozen yogurt or ice milk over layers, just as you would frosting. Work fairly quickly, so that you can finish before ice cream melts off cake. Freeze for several hours.

Fifteen minutes or so before serving, remove cake from freezer. Place berries and flags around top, if desired. Slice to serve.

YIELD: 16 servings

Each serving (1/16 of cake, with fat-free frozen yogurt): 187 calories, 0 g fat, (0% calories from fat), 0 g saturated fat, 0 g polyunsaturated fat, 0 g monounsaturated fat, 0 mg cholesterol, 43 g carbohydrate, 5 g protein, 171 mg sodium

EXCHANGES: 2 fruits, 1 bread

Apricot Cream Cake

◆

I don't use many boxed cake mixes or much Cool Whip, but this recipe was sent to me by a subscriber, Jane Johnson from Conyers, Georgia, and, after testing it, I decided it was perfect for the people who want a sinfully rich-tasting quick dessert.

You will not need all of the frosting mixture for this cake. Use it instead as a dip for fresh fruit or as a dressing for a fruit salad.

1 pkg. Pillsbury Loving Lites yellow cake mix

Filling:
1 c. sugar
1 carton (12 oz.) fat-free sour cream
1 jar (10–15 oz.) low-sugar apricot spread

Frosting:
1½ c. Lite Cool Whip
Optional: 1 can (15 oz.) apricot halves, drained, for
    garnish

Prepare cake according to package instructions. Bake in two 8- or 9-inch round cake pans. When cool, cut each layer in half horizontally so that you have four thin layers.

While cake is baking, prepare filling by combining sugar and fat-free sour cream. Chill the mixture.

When ready to assemble cake, set aside 1 cup sour cream mixture for frosting. Top each layer with remaining filling and then dot apricot spread evenly over filling.

Prepare frosting by combining the reserved 1 cup of sour cream mixture with Lite Cool Whip. Spread mixture over top and sides of cake. If desired, place drained apricot halves on top of cake in circle around outside edge.

Seal in airtight container and refrigerate. Tastes best after three days.

YIELD: 16 servings

Each serving (¹⁄₁₆ of cake): Approx. 223 calories, 2.1 g fat (8.5% calories from fat), 1 g saturated fat, 0.8 g polyunsaturated fat, 0 g monounsaturated fat, 5 g carbohydrate, 3 g protein, 223 mg sodium

EXCHANGES: 1 bread, 1½ fruits, ½ fat

"Un-Pound" Cake

◆

Judy Reisman of Washington, D.C., reports that this cake rates an A+ in the "disappearance factor." Of all the low-fat tub margarines I tested in this recipe, I found Weight Watchers Country Cottage Farms spread to give the nicest texture and a true buttery flavor. "Diet" margarines vary widely in their fat content. Before selecting one, be sure to read labels and compare the amount of fat per tablespoon.

1 tub (8 oz.) diet tub margarine
2 c. sugar
1 c. egg substitute
1 Tbsp. vanilla, brandy, lemon, orange, or almond extract
1 c. skim milk
3 c. flour
1 Tbsp. baking powder
Confectioners' sugar

Preheat oven to 350°F. Lightly coat 10-inch tube pan with vegetable oil spray.

Melt margarine, add sugar and egg substitute, and stir until smooth.

In one small bowl, mix flavor extract into milk. In another, stir together flour and baking powder. Stir milk mixture and flour mixture alternately into sugar-egg mixture. Batter will appear wetter than in a standard cake.

Bake about 50 minutes, or until cake tester comes out clean. When completely cooled, dust with confectioners' sugar and cover tightly.

YIELD: 24 servings

Each serving: 159 calories, 4.2 g fat (23.8% calories from fat), 1.3 g saturated fat, 0.7 g polyunsaturated, 0.6 g monounsaturated fat, 0 mg cholesterol, 28.2 g carbohydrate, 3.0 g protein, 66 mg sodium

EXCHANGES: 1 bread; 1 fruit; 1 fat

Creamy Cheesecake

◆

Never again should you feel guilty for eating this favorite. It is unbelievably thick and creamy with a distinctive cheesecake flavor—delicious when topped with fruit. Don't let the lengthy instructions intimidate you. They are included so that even a beginning cook can master this cheesecake on the first try.

I love *thick* cheesecake. This recipe makes a very generous cake, but it will be even thicker if you prepare it in an 8-inch round pan. If you don't have one, a 9-inch pan will work just as well, although the cake won't be as thick.

Step 1: Draining the Yogurt to Make Yogurt Cheese

    2 qt. plain nonfat yogurt (*must not contain gelatin*)

The night before, or eight hours before, making the cake, line a large colander with 2 layers of cheese-cloth. Set colander over large bowl, and scoop yogurt into colander. Cover bowl with dish towel, and refrigerate overnight or for 8 hours.

In the morning, remove the yogurt cheese from colander (you will have about 1 qt.), and discard the watery whey left in the bowl. Use the yogurt cheese immediately, or refrigerate until ready to use.

Step 2: Making the Cheesecake

    ½ c. graham cracker crumbs for 8½-inch pan; ¾ c. for
       larger pan
    2 pkg. (8 oz. ea.) light cream cheese
    2 eggs
    1 c. sugar

1 Tbsp. vanilla extract
2 Tbsp. cornstarch
Optional: ¼ tsp. salt
1 qt. yogurt cheese (see above)

Preheat oven to 350°F., and lightly coat bottom and
sides of springform pan, or 8- or 9-inch round cake
pan, with vegetable oil spray. Pour graham cracker
crumbs into pan, swirl pan so crumbs stick to sides,
and then distribute remaining crumbs evenly over bottom of pan. Make bottom of springform pan watertight
by covering outside of pan with wide heavy-duty aluminum foil.

Place cream cheese, eggs, sugar, vanilla extract,
cornstarch, and salt in bowl of food processor or
blender, and process until creamy smooth. Continue
with rest of recipe in the food processor, if possible.
Otherwise, transfer mixture to bowl, and proceed with
a mixer.

Add yogurt cheese, and process or mix until mixture is smooth and creamy. Use a cup measure to pour
mixture into prepared pan *gently* so as not to disturb
graham crackers. When all cheesecake mixture is in
pan, smooth top with rubber spatula. Place springform
pan in larger pan. Add water to outer pan until it is ½
inch to 1 inch from top of springform pan. Place pan
in oven, and bake 50 minutes.

Carefully remove pan from oven, and allow cheesecake pan to sit in hot water for 30 minutes. Then
remove springform pan from water and remove foil.
Cool 30 minutes longer at room temperature. Then
cover and refrigerate.

Serve cheesecake cold.

Y I E L D : 1 large cheesecake (16 servings)

Each serving: 208 calories, 6.3 g fat (26.7% calories from fat), 3.3 g saturated fat, 0.1 g polyunsaturated fat, 0.3 g monounsaturated fat, 46 mg cholesterol, 28 g carbohydrate, 11 g protein (1 serving contains 270 mg calcium, almost 33% of RDA; also an excellent source of protein and phosphorus

E X C H A N G E S : 1 skim milk; 1 bread; 1 fat

Chocolate Marble Cheesecake

—◆—

Here is a delicious low-fat cheesecake that tastes as good as it looks. I use an 8-inch springform pan for my cheesecakes, because it makes them thicker, but a standard 9-inch pan also works fine.

¼ c. graham cracker crumbs for 8-inch pan (½ c. for
   9-inch pan)
12 oz. fat-free Philadelphia cream cheese
2 eggs
1 c. plus ¼ c. sugar
3 Tbsp. cornstarch
Optional: ¼ tsp. salt
1 Tbsp. vanilla extract
32 oz. fat-free sour cream
¼ c. cocoa powder
2 Tbsp. skim milk
Optional: Chocolate syrup

Preheat oven to 350°F., and lightly coat springform pan with vegetable oil spray. Pour graham cracker crumbs into pan, swirl pan so crumbs stick to sides, and distribute remaining crumbs evenly over bottom of pan.

Place fat-free cream cheese, eggs, the 1 c. sugar, cornstarch, optional salt, and vanilla extract in bowl of food processor, and process until smooth and thick. Add fat-free sour cream, and process again until smooth, scraping sides of bowl, if necessary.

Measure out 1 cup of cheesecake mixture, and set aside. Pour rest into crust slowly until bottom is completely covered. Smooth top with spatula.

Stir together the cocoa powder, and the remaining ¼ c. sugar, and add to reserved cheesecake mixture along with the skim milk. Drop chocolate mixture on top of cheesecake, a tablespoonful at a time. Use knife to swirl chocolate through cheesecake, being careful not to cut all the way through to the crust, as that will cause crust to stir into cheesecake.

Bake 60 minutes, or until cooked through but not browned. Remove from oven and cool at room temperature 45–60 minutes. Cover and refrigerate until completely chilled (3–4 hours). If you wish, drizzle plate with small amount of chocolate syrup, like Hershey's, before placing cheesecake on plate.

YIELD: 16 servings

Each serving: 157 calories, 1.4 g fat (8.0% calories from fat), 0.4 g saturated fat, 0.2 g polyunsaturated fat, 0.5 g monounsaturated fat, 40 mg cholesterol, 26.1 g carbohydrate, 9.2 g protein, 223 mg sodium

EXCHANGES: 1 skim milk; 1 fruit

COOKIES

Chocolate Chip Cookies

◆

What childhood is complete without chocolate chip cookies hot from the oven? My cookie jar always has a ready supply of these for my two children and their friends—and for my husband, who has never fully outgrown his fondness for them! Full of whole wheat, and without the usual added fats, these are a healthful alternative to the old standard Toll-House cookies most of us remember from our childhood.

Cookies so low in fat do not keep well, but they usually don't stay around long enough for that to be a problem! Store them in a cookie jar; plastic containers and bags will cause them to soften.

    2 large eggs
    1 c. dark brown sugar
    ½ c. white sugar
    1 tsp. vanilla extract
    2 Tbsp. skim milk
    1 c. whole wheat flour
    1 c. white flour
    1 tsp. baking soda
    1 tsp. salt
    1 pkg. (12 oz.) chocolate chips

Preheat oven to 375°F., and lightly coat two cookie sheets with vegetable oil spray.

Beat together eggs, brown sugar, white sugar, vanilla, and skim milk until thick and uniformly mixed. Add whole wheat flour, white flour, baking soda, and salt, and beat again until well combined. Add more white flour, a tablespoon at a time, *if necessary,* beating after each addition, until mixture is no longer wet-looking and is thick enough not to run off the beater when beater is lifted from bowl. Add chocolate chips, and mix until chips are evenly distributed.

Drop dough onto cookie sheets by teaspoonfuls, leaving about 2 inches between cookies. Bake 8–10 minutes, or until only slightly browned and no longer wet when touched. Cookies will become hard if over-baked, so watch them carefully.

Cool 4–5 minutes on cookie sheets, and then transfer to rack.

YIELD: 36 two-inch cookies

Each cookie: 86 calories, 2.6 g fat (27.2% calories from fat), 1.4 g saturated fat, <0.1 g polyunsaturated fat, 0.1 g monounsaturated fat, 14 mg cholesterol, 15.6 g carbohydrate, 1.3 g protein, 91 mg sodium

EXCHANGES: ½ bread; ½ fruit; ½ fat

VARIATION: To make Chocolate Chip Cookies for Nut-Lovers, stir in ½ c. chopped pecans. This will add calories and fat to 91.5 calories (39% calories from fat) and 4.0 g fat per cookie. Yield will increase to 46 cookies.

VARIATION: For Extra-Low-Fat Cookies, use egg substitute instead of the eggs, and stir in only ½ pkg. (6 oz.) chips. Calories drop to 73.5 (17.1% calories from fat) and fat to 1.4 g. Yield will remain at 36 cookies.

Oatmeal-Raisin Cookies

◆

Credit for this recipe must go to my neighbor who called one night and asked me to come up with a low-fat oatmeal-raisin cookie. Never again will your children enjoy whole wheat flour and oatmeal as much as in this recipe, and at quite a fat savings from the original recipe!

¾ c. dark brown sugar
¼ c. white sugar
1 egg
1 tsp. vanilla extract
2 Tbsp. skim milk
1 c. oatmeal
½ c. all-purpose flour
½ c. whole wheat flour
½ tsp. baking soda
½ tsp. baking powder
½ tsp. salt
½ tsp. ground cinnamon
⅔ c. raisins or currants

Preheat oven to 375°F., and lightly coat two cookie sheets with vegetable oil spray.

In large bowl, mix together brown sugar, white sugar, and egg until thick and uniform, and then mix in vanilla extract and milk. In separate bowl, stir together oatmeal, all-purpose flour, whole wheat flour, baking soda, baking powder, salt, and cinnamon. Add flour mixture to egg-sugar mixture. When well combined, add raisins, and mix until evenly distributed.

Drop dough by teaspoonfuls onto cookie sheets, leaving about two inches between cookies. Bake 8–10 minutes, or until soft but firm throughout and slightly browned. Cool thoroughly on rack, and store in airtight container.

YIELD: 32 cookies

Each cookie: 61 calories, 0.4 g fat (5.9% calories from fat), 0.1 g saturated fat, <0.1 g polyunsaturated fat, <0.1 g monounsaturated fat, 9 mg cholesterol, 13.8 g carbohydrate, 1.1 g protein, 61 mg sodium

EXCHANGES: 1 bread

Gingersnaps

◆

These cookies are so good that most people will agree that they don't need fat. Use more or less ginger, cinnamon, and nutmeg depending on the amount of spiciness you like best.

2 eggs
1½ c. sugar
¾ c. molasses
1 tsp. cider vinegar
2 c. all-purpose flour
1½ c. whole wheat flour
1½ tsp. baking soda
1 Tbsp. grated fresh ginger or ground ginger
½ tsp. ground cinnamon
¼ tsp. ground nutmeg

Preheat oven to 325°F., and lightly coat cookie sheets with vegetable oil spray.

In large bowl, beat together the eggs, sugar, molasses, and vinegar. In smaller bowl, mix remaining ingredients, and add them to egg-molasses mixture. Beat just until well combined.

Drop by teaspoonfuls onto cookie sheets 3 or 4 inches apart. Bake 8–10 minutes for chewy cookies, or 12–13 minutes for crispier ones (until slightly brown).

Cool to room temperature on rack. Store in airtight container, or freeze for up to 1 month.

YIELD: Approx. 72 cookies

Each cookie: 46 calories, 0.2 g fat (3.9% calories from fat), <0.1 g saturated fat, <0.1 g polyunsaturated fat, <0.1 g monounsaturated fat, 8 mg cholesterol, 10.5 g carbohydrate, 0.8 g protein, 29 mg sodium

EXCHANGES: ½ bread

Choco-Nut Cranberry Cookies

2 eggs
1 c. dark brown sugar, packed
½ c. white granulated sugar
1 tsp. vanilla extract
2 Tbsp. skim milk
2¼ c. all-purpose flour
1 tsp. baking soda
1 tsp. salt
6 oz. chocolate chips
½ c. coarsely chopped cranberries
½ c. whole almonds, shelled

Preheat oven to 375°F., and lightly coat cookie sheets with vegetable oil spray.

In large bowl, beat together eggs, brown sugar, and white sugar until thick and very smooth. Add vanilla extract and skim milk, beating again until smooth. Combine flour, baking soda, and salt in separate bowl, stirring with spoon until well mixed. Add flour mixture to egg mixture, and beat until dough is thick and all dry ingredients are wet. Stir in chocolate chips, cranberries, and almonds until uniformly combined.

Drop by teaspoonfuls onto cookie sheets. Bake 8–10 minutes, until lightly browned and only slightly damp in center. Cool 5 minutes on cookie sheet, then transfer to rack. When completely cool, store at room temperature in sealed plastic bags.

YIELD: 40 cookies

Each cookie: 96 calories, 3.0 g fat (28% calories from fat), 1.1 g saturated fat, 0.3 g polyunsaturated fat, 1.0 g mono- unsaturated fat, 14 mg cholesterol, 15.9 g carbohydrate, 1.8 g protein, 91 mg sodium

EXCHANGES: 1 bread

Chocolate Fudge Brownies

There are almost as many ideas of a perfect brownie as there are brownie lovers, but here is a low-fat version that is a wonderful start.

Use your favorite cocoa powder in this recipe. If you don't have a favorite, Hershey makes two different kinds. Their

European-style cocoa, which comes in a silver tin, makes a
brownie that is dark and rich, while their regular cocoa, in
the brown tin, produces medium dark brownies with a sharp
but less complex chocolate flavor. My family's favorite is the
European-style, but use whichever you prefer.

½ c. unsweetened cocoa powder
1¼ c. cake flour, lightly spooned into cup
1½ c. sugar
½ tsp. baking powder
½ tsp. salt
⅓ c. water
2 eggs or substitute egg equivalent
1 tsp. vanilla extract

Preheat oven to 350°F., and lightly coat 8-inch-square
pan with vegetable oil spray.

In large bowl, whisk together cocoa powder, flour,
sugar, baking powder, and salt until mixture is very
smooth and no clumps remain. In separate bowl,
whisk together water, eggs, and vanilla extract until
well combined. Add egg mixture to dry ingredients,
mixing only until all flour disappears and mixture is
smooth. Batter will be thick.

Pour batter into pan, and spread evenly. Bake 25–30
minutes, or until brownies are no longer wet but are
still moist when gently pushed in center of pan. Do
not overbake.

Cool brownies completely before cutting. Clean
knife during cutting, if necessary.

YIELD: 16 brownies

Each brownie: 121 calories, 1.1 g fat (8.4% calories from
fat), 0.2 g saturated fat, <0.1 g polyunsaturated fat, 0.3 g

monounsaturated fat, 34 mg cholesterol, 26 g carbohydrate, 2 g protein, 50 mg sodium

EXCHANGES: 1 bread; 1 fruit

VARIATION: For Cakelike Brownies, increase flour to 1½ c. and add ½ c. water.

OTHER DESSERTS

Apple Bundles

———◆———

Here's a beautiful dessert worthy of your most special occasions.

    24 sheets phyllo dough
    1 Tbsp. vegetable oil
    4 large cooking apples, peeled, cored, and very thinly
        sliced
    ¼ c. sugar
    ¼ c. raisins
    ½ tsp. ground cinnamon
    Confectioners' sugar
    3 Tbsp. honey

Preheat oven to 350°F. Spray a large baking sheet lightly with vegetable oil spray. Unroll sheets of phyllo dough to one stack of flat sheets, and cut about 8 inches from one end so that sheets are 8 inches shorter. Cover dough with damp cloth to keep it from drying out. Have rest of ingredients ready.

Lay two sheets of phyllo dough, one on top of the other, on work surface. Brush a very thin layer of oil over the dough, and place third sheet on top, lining up all corners. Place one-eighth of apples (slices from one-half apple) on middle of top phyllo sheet. Top with ½ Tbsp. sugar, ½ Tbsp. raisins, and a sprinkle of cinnamon. Pull all four corners of dough up over apples. Secure dough by tying string loosely around juncture (see diagram), and place bundle on large

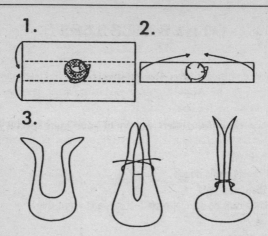

baking sheet. Repeat for all bundles. (They may be immediately frozen at this point for 1–2 days.)

When all bundles are assembled (or immediately after removing them from freezer), bake 15 minutes (25 minutes if frozen), or until bundles are medium brown and dough is baked and crispy.

To serve, sprinkle confectioners' sugar lightly over top of each, and drizzle 1 tsp. honey onto each bundle. Serve hot.

YIELD: 8 bundles

Each bundle: 199 calories, 2.4 g fat (10.9% calories from fat), 0.3 g saturated fat, 1.4 g polyunsaturated fat, 0.4 g monounsaturated fat, 4 mg cholesterol, 47.8 g carbohydrate, 2.6 g protein, 68 mg sodium

EXCHANGES: 2 fruits; 1 bread; ½ fat

Fresh Peach Cobbler

---◆---

If you like cobblers, you'll enjoy this recipe. Instructions are also given for an Apple Cobbler variation, since peaches are in season for such a short time.

You can bake this dessert in an oblong pan (8 by 12 inches), if you wish. Just make 1½ times the amount of topping in the recipe.

15 ripe medium-size peaches, peeled and sliced
½ c. sugar
½ tsp. ground cinnamon
¼ c. water
¼ c. water mixed with 2 Tbsp. cornstarch

Topping:
1 c. all-purpose flour
2 tsp. baking powder
Pinch salt
¼ c. plus 3 Tbsp. sugar
¼ c. fat-free sour cream
¼ c. plus 2 Tbsp. skim milk

Preheat oven to 350°F. Place peaches, ½ c. sugar, cinnamon, and the ¼ c. plain water in large heavy saucepan. Bring to a boil, stir, and reduce heat to medium. Cook 5–10 minutes, until peaches are moderately tender, and then add the ¼ c. water mixed with 2 Tbsp. cornstarch. Bring to a boil, and cook until thickened.

While peaches are cooking, prepare the topping. Stir together flour, baking powder, salt, and the ¼ c. sugar. Add the fat-free sour cream and all of the milk, and stir until well combined.

When peaches are thoroughly cooked, pour them and their liquid into an ungreased 8-inch-square baking pan. Drop the topping, a tablespoon at a time, onto top of peaches. With back of spoon, spread topping so that it covers most of the filling. Sprinkle remaining 3 Tbsp. sugar evenly over surface, and bake cobbler 20 minutes, or until topping is browned and dessert is cooked through.

YIELD: 12 servings

Each serving: 152 calories, 0.2 g fat (1.2% calories from fat), <0.1 g saturated fat, <0.1 g polyunsaturated fat, <0.1 g monounsaturated fat, <0.1 mg cholesterol, 36.7 g carbohydrate, 2.6 g protein, 50 mg sodium

EXCHANGES: 1 bread; 1½ fruits

VARIATION: For Apple Cobbler, substitute 10 medium Granny Smith apples for the peaches, and omit the cornstarch. Cook only 5 minutes after mixture reaches a boil.

Lemon Meringue Pie

◆

Meringue is fat-free, and it makes a beautiful topping for low-fat desserts. Long before I started school, I loved watching my grandmother and her friends baking and cooling their meringue-topped pies and taking pride in the tallest and prettiest. Here is a low-fat version of the traditional summertime lemon meringue pie.

¼ c. graham cracker crumbs
1 c. sugar
6 Tbsp. cornstarch
Optional: ¼ tsp. salt
2 egg yolks (save whites for meringue)
2¼ c. cold water
½ c. freshly squeezed lemon juice (about 3 medium-
   large lemons)
1 Tbsp. lemon zest
Lemon zest strips or thin slices of lemon for garnish

Meringue:
3 egg whites
¼ tsp. cream of tartar
3 Tbsp. sugar
½ tsp. vanilla extract

Preheat oven to 350°F., and lightly coat 9-inch pie plate with vegetable oil spray. Pour graham cracker crumbs into pie plate, and swirl so that crumbs stick to sides. Distribute rest of crumbs evenly over bottom of plate.

In small saucepan, stir together the 1 c. sugar, cornstarch, and optional salt. Whisk in the egg yolks until thick and well-mixed. Add water, lemon juice, and lemon zest. Place saucepan over medium-high heat, and bring to a boil, stirring constantly. When thickened, pour lemon mixture, a tablespoon at a time at first so not to disturb the crust, into pie plate. Smooth surface with spatula.

To make meringue, place egg whites in mixing bowl, and mix on medium speed until whites become frothy. Add cream of tartar, and beat at highest speed until whites begin to stiffen. Add the 3 Tbsp. sugar, a tablespoon at a time, and continue beating until whites are glossy and hold stiff peaks when beater is lifted. Add vanilla extract and beat 10 seconds more. Spread meringue evenly over top of lemon filling, pulling meringue to sides of dish. Use knife to swirl meringue, making pretty peaks over surface. Bake 10 minutes, or until lightly browned and cooked through.

Remove from oven. Cool at room temperature until cooled (30–45 minutes), and then cover lightly with plastic wrap and refrigerate several hours. Garnish with long strips of lemon zest or thin slices of lemon.

YIELD: 12 servings

Each serving (1/12 of pie): 112 calories, 1.1 g fat (8.8% calories from fat), 0.3 g saturated fat, 0.1 g polyunsaturated fat, 0.4 g monounsaturated fat, 46 mg cholesterol, 24.7 g carbohydrate, 1.5 g protein, 75 mg sodium

EXCHANGES: 1 fruit; 1 bread

Chocolate Belgian Waffles

◆

Here's a dessert for chocolate lovers! Since these are most impressive and delicious served warm, make up the batter three or four hours ahead, place in the refrigerator, and cook right before serving.

If you do not have a Belgian waffle iron, use a regular iron. A regular waffle iron will make a larger quantity of smaller waffles.

½ c. unsweetened cocoa powder
1½ c. cake flour
1 c. sugar
½ tsp. baking powder
½ tsp. baking soda
¼ tsp. salt
1 egg
¾ c. water
1 tsp. vanilla extract
1 Tbsp. vegetable oil
Optional: 6 dollops Lite Cool Whip

Preheat waffle iron and lightly coat cooking surfaces with vegetable oil spray.

In large mixing bowl, whisk together the cocoa powder, flour, sugar, baking powder, baking soda, and salt. In smaller bowl, mix together the egg, water, vanilla extract, and oil until egg is well dispersed.

Add egg mixture to dry ingredients, and stir with wooden spoon just until all flour is mixed in and large clumps disappear. Pour manufacturer's recommended amount of batter onto grids of Belgian waffle iron. Cook 1½ to 2 minutes, until firm but now browned.

Serve while warm, topped with dollop of Lite Cool Whip, if you wish.

YIELD: 6 large Belgian waffles, or more smaller waffles, depending on waffle iron used

Each large Belgian waffle: 279 calories, 4.4 g fat (14.1% calories from fat), 0.6 g saturated fat, 1.4 g polyunsaturated fat, 0.9 g monounsaturated fat, 51 mg cholesterol, 21 g carbohydrate, 5 g protein, 228 mg sodium

EXCHANGES: 1½ breads; 1 fat

Mincemeat Bread Pudding with Rum Sauce

◆

Here's a dessert for anyone who loves the flavor of mincemeat but finds mincemeat pie a bit too much—and too fatty! If you start the mincemeat when you begin soaking the bread cubes in milk, your timing should be perfect. Serve this dessert as soon as you remove it from the oven, if possible, because, like a souffle, it loses volume somewhat when it cools.

4 c. stale bread cubes
3 c. skim milk
¼ tsp. salt
2 eggs
½ c. sugar
1 tsp. vanilla extract
1 c. diced apples
1 c. raisins
1 c. golden raisins
½ c. dark brown sugar
1 c. water
1 tsp. ground cinnamon
1 tsp. ground allspice
½ tsp. ground nutmeg
2 tsp. rum extract
1 c. water
1½ tsp. rum extract
⅓ c. sugar
¼ tsp. ground cinnamon
1½ Tbsp. cornstarch mixed with 2 Tbsp. water

Combine the bread cubes, skim milk, salt, eggs, ½ c. sugar, and vanilla extract in a large bowl. Leave to sit at room temperature until mincemeat mixture below has cooked.

Stir together the apples, raisins, golden raisins, brown sugar, 1 c. water, spices, and rum extract in a heavy saucepan. Bring to a boil. Simmer about 30 minutes. Turn off heat, and let mixture sit for at least another 30 minutes.

Preheat oven to 350°F. Lightly coat 10-inch-square baking pan with vegetable oil spray.

Stir mincemeat mixture into the soaking bread cubes, and pour into prepared pan. Bake for 45–60 minutes, or until pudding has risen and is set in middle.

While pudding is baking, prepare rum sauce. Combine 1 c. water, rum, sugar, cinnamon, and cornstarch/water mixture in a small saucepan. Heat, stirring constantly. When sauce begins to boil and is thickened and clear, remove from heat.

Serve hot pudding topped with rum sauce.

YIELD: 12 servings

Each serving: 209 calories, 1.7 g fat (7.3% calories from fat), 0.5 g saturated fat, <0.1 g polyunsaturated fat, 0.6 g monounsaturated fat, 47 mg cholesterol, 45.0 g carbohydrate, 4.9 g protein, 157 mg sodium

EXCHANGES: 2 breads; 1 fruit

Rice Pudding

◆

Here is an old-fashioned dessert, often thought of as a comfort food. It's probably best prepared with arborio rice (an Italian rice), but any short-grain rice will do. I often use Turkish or Egyptian rice, since it is inexpensive and available in the Asian groceries in the Washington, D.C., area.

Sometimes I use a tip from the *New Basics Cookbook* (Julee Rosso and Sheila Lukins, 1989, p. 752): I soak the raisins in Frangelico liqueur while the pudding is cooking and then add them to the pudding at the end. Yum!

⅓ c. short-grain rice
4 c. skim milk
⅓ c. sugar
½ c. raisins or currants
1 tsp. vanilla extract
Optional: Berries or other fruits
Optional: Ground cinnamon or nutmeg

Combine rice, milk, and sugar in top of double boiler. Place over simmering water, and stir every 10 minutes or so for 1 hour, or until rice is tender and most of milk has been absorbed. Add raisins or currants during last 10 minutes of cooking (or at the end, if they were soaked in liqueur). Let pudding cool 15–20 minutes, and then stir in vanilla extract.

Serve warm or cold. If desired, serve topped with berries or other fruit, or with a sprinkling of ground cinnamon or nutmeg.

YIELD: 6 servings

Each serving: 143 calories, 0.4 g fat (2.5% calories from fat), 0.2 g saturated fat, <0.1 g polyunsaturated fat, <0.1 g monounsaturated fat, 3 mg cholesterol, 28.6 g carbohydrate, 6.4 g protein, 84 mg sodium

EXCHANGES: 2 breads

Frozen Fruit Salad

◆

I prefer to use Dannon or Columbo nonfat yogurt in this frozen salad. I love to serve it for dessert on hot summer days. Use your own fresh fruit mixture if you have time to prepare it.

1 can (16 oz.) fruit cocktail packed in juice or extra-light
    syrup, drained
1 can (11 oz.) mandarin orange segments, drained and
    broken up
2 bananas, chopped
1½ c. vanilla nonfat yogurt
Fresh mint or orange slices for garnish

Mix together all ingredients except mint or orange-slice garnish. Pour into loaf pan, and freeze until firm.

Remove from freezer, and let sit at room temperature for about 15 minutes before serving. Cut into ¾-inch-thick slices, and top with fresh mint or orange slice.

YIELD: 12 servings

Each serving: 86 calories, 0.2 g fat (2.1% calories from fat), <0.1 g saturated fat, <0.1 g polyunsaturated fat, <0.1

monounsaturated fat, <1 mg cholesterol, 10.0 g carbohydrate, 2.2 g protein, 23 mg sodium

EXCHANGES: ½ fruit; ¼ skim milk

Raspberry Bavarian Cream

---◆---

This delightful fruit dessert can be made quickly. If you use sweetened berries, omit the sugar in the recipe.

    1 pkg. (10 oz.) unsweetened frozen raspberries
    2 pkg. (¼ oz. each) unflavored gelatin
    ½ c. sugar
    1 can (12 oz.) evaporated skim milk
    ½ tsp. vanilla extract
    Optional: Lite Cool Whip

Set sieve over bowl, pour berries into sieve, and allow juice to drain into bowl for at least 30 minutes.

After berries have drained, measure raspberry juice in bowl. Add water, if necessary, to make ⅔ cup. Pour gelatin into juice, and stir to eliminate large clumps. Let mixture stand 3–5 minutes until gelatin is softened, and then stir in sugar.

Bring juice and gelatin mixture to a boil in microwave (2–3 minutes), or in saucepan on burner. Stir very well, and cool to room temperature.

Beat evaporated skimmed milk in chilled bowl until thickened. Add cooled juice to milk in steady stream, and beat just until well combined. Pour into 8 wineglasses or into one large bowl. If desired, gently add half of berries to mixture as you are spooning dessert into glasses, but be sure to save some berries for topping. Refrigerate until mixture is well chilled.

Serve in wineglasses, or dip portions from large bowl into individual dishes. Serve topped with reserved raspberries and, if desired, 1 tablespoon Lite Cool Whip.

YIELD: 10 servings

Each ¾ cup serving = 75 calories, 0.1 g fat (1.7% calories from fat), <0.1 g saturated fat, <0.1 g polyunsaturated fat, <0.1 g monounsaturated fat, 1 mg cholesterol, 16 g carbohydrate, 3 g protein, 45 mg sodium

EXCHANGES: ½ skim milk; ½ fruit

Berry Shortcake

◆

Shortcake was traditionally made with sweetened biscuits rather than the sponge cakes now sold in supermarkets. Unlike true shortcake, this recipe uses no added fat, but it does yield a soft, biscuitlike base. This dessert can be made with fresh or frozen strawberries, blueberries, or blackberries. Canned blueberries and blackberries also work well.

1 c. all-purpose flour
1½ tsp. baking powder
Pinch salt
2 Tbsp. sugar
¼ c. fat-free sour cream
6 Tbsp. unsweetened applesauce
¼ c. skim milk

Optional: 1½ tsp. sugar

3 c. sliced strawberries, or 3 c. whole blackberries
   or blueberries

Optional: 2 Tbsp. sugar

1 c. fat-free vanilla yogurt

Preheat oven to 350°F., and lightly coat baking sheet
with vegetable oil spray. Combine flour, baking powder, salt, and sugar. Stir in fat-free sour cream, applesauce, and milk, and mix only until flour is all
combined. Drop by tablespoonfuls onto baking sheet,
dividing it into six servings. If desired, sprinkle the 1½
tsp. sugar over the shortcakes, using about ¼ tsp. on
each cake. Bake 20 minutes, or until lightly browned
and cooked through. Transfer to rack to cool.

Sweeten berries with the remaining 2 Tbsp. sugar,
if desired.

Place 1 shortcake on each dessert plate, and top
with ½ c. fruit and dollop of vanilla yogurt.

YIELD: 6 servings

Each serving: 161 calories, 0.6 g fat (3.3% calories from
fat), 0.1 g saturated fat, 0.2 g polyunsaturated fat, 0.1 g
monounsaturated fat, 1 mg cholesterol, 33.2 g carbohydrate,
6.1 g protein, 151 mg sodium

EXCHANGES: 1 bread; 1 fruit

Raspberry-Pear Compote

———— ◆ ————

3 cans (16 oz. each) light pear halves in juice
2 pkgs. (10 oz. each) frozen whole raspberries in light
   syrup
½ Tbsp. cornstarch mixed with 1 Tbsp. water

Drain pears and raspberries, reserving ¾ c. of their juice. Mix together reserved raspberry and pear juice in small heavy saucepan. Spoon half of the raspberries into a sieve, place sieve over saucepan, and use back of spoon to press as much juice as possible from the berries into juice mixture. Discard pulp and seeds left in sieve. Bring juice to a boil, and reduce to half its original volume (5–10 minutes). Reduce heat, add cornstarch mixture, and cook slowly until thickened.

To assemble compote, place 2 or 3 pear halves in bottom of each of 8 large wine goblets. Top pear halves with raspberries. Drizzle syrup lightly over each compote.

YIELD: 8 servings

Each serving: 154 calories, 0.2 g fat (1.2% calories from fat), <0.1 g saturated fat, 0.1 g polyunsaturated fat, <0.1 g monounsaturated fat, 0 mg cholesterol, 37 g carbohydrate, 1 g protein, 4 mg sodium

EXCHANGES: 2½ fruits

Orange Sections with Grand Marnier

◆

Sometimes the simplest desserts can be the most enjoyable. Here's one that's refreshing, especially after a heavy meal. (Leave the Grand Marnier out of the children's portions.) This tastes best when made with California navel oranges, but you may add other seasonal fruits for color.

2–4 Tbsp. Grand Marnier, to taste
4 large or 8 small navel oranges, peeled and separated
    into sections

In large bowl, pour Grand Marnier over fruit. Toss well, and set aside at room temperature for at least 30 minutes, tossing occasionally. Serve in 6 pretty stemmed goblets.

YIELD: 6 servings

Each serving: 80 calories, 0 g fat (0% calories from fat), 0 g saturated fat, 0 g polyunsaturated fat, 0 g monounsaturated fat, 0 mg cholesterol, 18 g carbohydrate, 0 g protein, 0 mg sodium

EXCHANGES: 1 fruit

Fruit Purees

◆

You'll find a lot of uses for fruit purees. Layer a puree with plain yogurt or ice milk in a stemmed glass for an easy but pretty dessert. Stir a puree into yogurt, or use one as a fruit sauce over angel food cake or waffles.

To make a simple sorbet, place 3 c. fruit puree in 8-inch-square baking pan or similar-size dish, cover with plastic wrap, and set in freezer. Stir puree after about 1 hour, and then freeze until solid. Remove from freezer and let sit at room temperature 5–10 minutes before spooning into dessert dishes.

4 c. fresh fruit, cut into 1-inch chunks
Optional: 2–4 Tbsp. sugar, to taste

Process fruit in blender or food processor until smooth, adding small amounts of water if necessary to produce the consistency you desire. When smooth, add sugar to taste, if you wish.

YIELD: Approx. 3 c. puree

Each ¼ c. serving: Approx. 30 calories, 0 g fat, (0% calories from fat), 0 g saturated fat, 0 g polyunsaturated fat, 0 g monounsaturated fat, 0 mg cholesterol, 8 g carbohydrate, 0 g protein

EXCHANGES: ½ fruit

Suggested Fruits:
Raspberries (fresh or frozen)
Strawberry-banana (about ½ and ½)
Fresh peaches
Fresh pineapple

Almond Biscotti

◆

These Italian cookies have become all the craze with espresso lovers, but they taste equally as good with tea and regular coffee. This remarkably easy recipe is low in fat because it is flavored with almond extract rather than almonds, although it does contain a few almonds for texture.

2¼ c. all-purpose flour
1½ tsp. baking powder
¼ tsp. salt
½ c. sugar
½ c. honey
2 eggs
1 tsp. almond extract
Zest of 1 lemon
¼ c. sliced almonds

Preheat oven to 350°F., and line a large baking sheet with parchment.

In one bowl, mix together flour, baking powder, salt, and sugar. In separate bowl, combine honey, eggs, almond extract, lemon zest, and almonds. Add the egg mixture to the dry ingredients, and mix until all ingredients are well incorporated.

Lay half of dough lengthwise on one side of parchment-lined baking sheet. Shape with hands into smooth log about 12 inches long, 4 inches wide, and ½ to ¾ inch thick. Shape remaining dough into second log parallel to the first, leaving at least four inches between the two.

Bake logs 20–30 minutes, until firm and medium brown. Remove from oven, and immediately cut into

¼-inch to ½-inch diagonal slices, using sharp serrated bread knife.

Reduce oven temperature to 300°F. Lay slices on baking sheet and bake 8–10 minutes, until lightly browned on one side. Flip cookies over, and bake 8–10 minutes longer. Remove from oven when firm. Cool on rack, and store in sealable plastic bag or airtight container.

YIELD: 50 cookies

Each cookie: 46 calories, 0.9 g fat (17.0% calories from fat), 0.1 g saturated fat, 0.2 g polyunsaturated fat, 0.5 g monounsaturated fat, 11 mg cholesterol, 8.8 g carbohydrate, 1.0 g protein, 21 mg sodium,

EXCHANGES: ½ bread

Fruit Kebabs
———◆———

Children love to eat food served on skewers. Let them choose their favorite fruits and arrange them in their own special pattern. Use this as an opportunity to encourage them to think about variety of flavor and color and to try some new fruits.

You'll need one wooden skewer for each person. These can be found in the cookout section of most grocery and department stores.

Assorted fruits, cut into bite-size chunks: melons,
    grapes, pineapple, apples, peaches, berries, plums,
    bananas dipped in orange or lemon juice
¼ c. dip: nonfat sour cream, Lite Cool Whip, vanilla or
    fruit-flavored fat-free yogurt, plain fat-free yogurt

mixed with small amount honey, or confectioners'
sugar

Push fruit onto skewers. Place skewers on salad-sized
plate along with ¼ c. dip. To eat, push fruit off skewer
with fork or fingers, and eat as is or with dip.

**Each serving: Approx. 60 calories, 0 g fat (0% calories from
fat), 0 g saturated fat, 0 g polyunsaturated fat, 0 g monounsaturated fat, 0 mg cholesterol, 0 g carbohydrate, 0 g protein,
0 mg sodium**

EXCHANGES: 1 fruit

Chocolate Chip Ice Cream Sandwiches

──────◆──────

**This informal treat is a perfect snack or outdoor dessert. It
may seem sinful, but it's really quite low in fat.**

2 chocolate chip cookies (page 247)
¼ c. vanilla or chocolate nonfat frozen yogurt

Place 1 scoop frozen yogurt on back of one cookie.
Top with second cookie, and press gently to make
sandwich.

YIELD: 1 sandwich

**Each sandwich: 197 calories, 5.2 g fat (23.8% calories from
fat), 2.8 g saturated fat, 0.1 g polyunsaturated fat, 0.2 g
monounsaturated fat, 28 mg cholesterol, 34.2 g carbohydrate,
3.6 g protein, 202 mg sodium**

EXCHANGES: 2 breads; 1 fat

Old-Fashioned "Ice Cream" Floats

————◆————

My family has recently rediscovered this delightful old-fashioned dessert. Don't limit yourself to the variations listed. Instead, use them as a starting point for creating your own masterpiece! Serve them with iced tea spoons and long straws.

½ cup nonfat frozen yogurt
Diet soda

Place frozen yogurt in tall glass, and add soda to fill glass.

YIELD: 1 serving

Each serving: Approx. 110 calories, 0 g fat (0% calories from fat), 0 g saturated fat, 0 g polyunsaturated fat, 0 g monounsaturated fat, 0 mg cholesterol, 25 g carbohydrate, 2 g protein, 50 mg sodium

EXCHANGES: 1½ bread

VARIATIONS: vanilla frozen yogurt with Diet Coke; pineapple-coconut sherbet with diet ginger ale; strawberry frozen yogurt with 7-Up, topped with chopped strawberries

Accompaniments

$\blacklozenge$

Having grown up with southern cooking, I find that it's very natural to use pickles, jams, and jellies as an accompaniment to simple meals. They can also be used hot, as a topping for sliced meats or plain vegetables.

Most pickles, jams, and fruit butters are made with little or no added fat. Here are a few of my personal favorites. Feel free to double or triple these recipes so that you'll have plenty to last all year as well as some to share with friends and family.

Fat-Free Cream Sauce

$\blacklozenge$

Here's a new recipe for fat-free cream sauce: Mix together 1 Tbsp. flour in 1 c. skim milk. Heat until thickened, and then season to taste with salt, pepper, dried bouillon, herbs, caraway seeds or toasted sesame seeds, mustard, garlic, and onion, chopped vegetables, or small amounts of low-fat cheese. Use more flour for a thicker sauce, less for a thinner one.

Tomato Chutney

$\blacklozenge$

When I recently brought this chutney to a local cooking class, it received rave reviews, even from people who don't normally like chutney. Use it with Indian food or serve it as a sauce over fish or chicken. Make extra chutney for gifts.

1 can (28 oz.) crushed tomatoes or 4 c. fresh chopped
  tomatoes
1 head garlic, all cloves peeled and chopped
3 Tbsp. minced fresh ginger
3 c. cider vinegar
2 c. sugar
Optional: ¼ tsp. ground red pepper or cayenne
¼ c. raisins or currants
2 Tbsp. sliced almonds

Combine tomatoes, garlic, ginger, vinegar, and sugar in heavy two-quart saucepan. Bring to a boil, and reduce heat to low. Simmer, uncovered, 45 minutes, or until mixture reaches the consistency of ketchup. Taste and add red pepper if desired. Stir in raisins or currants and almonds, and simmer 5–10 minutes longer.

Pour into glass pint jars, and refrigerate. Use within 1–2 months. To keep at room temperature, boil chutney and seal as you would jam or preserves.

YIELD: Approx. 3–4 cups

Each 1 Tbsp. serving: 35 calories, 0.3 g fat (7.8% calories from fat), <0.1 g saturated fat, <0.1 g polyunsaturated fat, 0.2 g monounsaturated fat, 0 mg cholesterol, 8.4 g carbohydrate, 0.4 g protein, 27 mg sodium

EXCHANGES: ½ fruit

Hot Pepper Jelly

◆

The first time I ever made this, I was surprised at how simple it was to prepare. Serve it atop low-fat cream cheese on crackers or, as I do, on plain toast.

If you can only locate green chili peppers, go ahead and use them, but substitute red bell peppers for the green.

You can grind the seeded peppers in a food processor, if you like, but rinse them thoroughly in a colander after grinding if they develop a milky-looking juice.

2 c. ground seeded green bell peppers
½–⅔ c. ground seeded red hot chili peppers
7½ c. sugar
1½ c. white vinegar
1 box (1¾ oz.) fruit pectin

Combine bell peppers, hot peppers, sugar, vinegar, and pectin in large, heavy pot. Bring mixture to a rolling boil, and continue to boil for 10 minutes. Immediately pour into sterilized jars, and seal. Invert jars on counter for 30 minutes or longer, and then turn right side up. Wait 1 hour; if any jars did not seal, boil them in hot water bath, or refrigerate them. Tastes best after a few days.

YIELD: 3 pints

Each 1 tsp. serving: Approx. 16 calories, 0 g fat (0% calories from fat), 0 g saturated fat, 0 g polyunsaturated fat, 0 g monounsaturated fat, 0 mg cholesterol, 4 g carbohydrate, 0 g protein, 2 mg sodium

EXCHANGES: ¼ fruit

Apple Butter

◆

Despite its name, apple butter doesn't contain any fat, but it certainly tastes good in place of butter on hot toast. It's good, too, used in place of applesauce in muffins. Just be sure to adjust the spices in your muffin recipe accordingly.

This recipe came to me from a neighbor, Russ Fyock. It was handwritten on an old piece of onionskin paper by his aunt, who made it from applesauce, which makes it fast and easy. It's a wonderful recipe to make use of when you need small hostess or holiday gifts.

A word of caution: Apple butter will "pop" as it cooks. *Always* keep the lid on the pot (but slightly ajar so steam can escape) to prevent the sauce from escaping. Use caution when you remove the lid to stir the sauce, and replace the lid immediately after stirring.

2 No. 10 cans unsweetened applesauce
1 jar (12 oz.) molasses
4–6 Tbsp. ground cinnamon
1 Tbsp. ground allspice
1 Tbsp. ground nutmeg
Optional: Additional sugar to taste
Optional: 1 tsp. salt

Combine all ingredients in heavy pot large enough so that applesauce does not fill it more than halfway. Bring mixture to a boil. Reduce heat, and simmer, covered (but open just enough to let steam escape), 3–4 hours, or until darkened and thick. *Take care not to let sauce splatter as it cooks.* Pour boiling apple butter into sterilized jars and seal. Check seals, and boil any unsealed jars for 10 minutes. Then recheck seal. (If you are unfamiliar with canning and making jams, read instructions in basic cookbook.)

YIELD: 10 or more pints

Each 1 Tbsp. serving: 10 calories, <0.1 g fat (1.2% calories from fat), 0 g saturated fat, 0 g polyunsaturated fat, 0 g monounsaturated fat, 0 mg cholesterol, 2.7 g carbohydrate, <0.1 g protein, <1 mg sodium

EXCHANGES: ⅕ fruit

Spiced Pickled Peaches

◆

My grandmother always had pickled peaches on her table during the winter holidays, and so do I. Since they are hard to find in the stores, I make my own during the summer when I can find fresh peaches at an affordable price. Be sure to make enough for gifts, as they are unusual and quite a conversation piece.

2 qt. plus 1 pt. water
1 Tbsp. salt
1 Tbsp. plus 1 pt. cider vinegar
5 pounds small fresh peaches, ripe but still firm
6 c. sugar
2 cinnamon sticks, broken up
1 Tbsp. whole cloves

Wash and sterilize five or six 1-pint jars. If you are unfamiliar with canning, read canning instructions in a basic cookbook.

Place the 2 quarts water, the salt, and the 1 Tbsp.

vinegar in large pot, and stir until salt is dissolved. Set aside.

Fill separate large stockpot or canning kettle about halfway with water, and bring to a boil. Add peaches, several at a time, to boiling water, and boil for about 1 minute. Use slotted spoon to transfer peaches to sink filled with very cold water. When peaches are cool enough to handle, peel them. (Skins should come off easily.) Drop peeled peaches into the salt water and vinegar solution in first kettle, to prevent them from turning brown.

In large pot, combine the 1 pt. vinegar, the 1 pt. water, and the sugar, cinnamon, and cloves, and heat mixture until sugar dissolves. Add peaches—in two or three batches, if necessary—and simmer in syrup 5–10 minutes, or until just tender. Do not overcook, or peaches will begin to fall apart.

Use slotted spoon to remove spices from pot. (Discard spices.) Fill jar with cooked peaches, packing them loosely to within 1 inch of top. Ladle juice from kettle to within ½ inch of top. Wipe off rim and seal jar. Repeat until 5 or 6 jars are filled. Then heat jars in hot water bath, remove them, and check seals. Store in dark pantry or closet. Best after 1–2 months.

YIELD: **Approx. 5 pt.**

Each peach: approx. 79 calories, 0.1 g fat (1.1% calories from fat), <0.1 g saturated fat, <0.1 g polyunsaturated fat, <0.1 g monounsaturated fat, 0 mg cholesterol, 20.5 g carbohydrate, 0.5 g protein, 22 mg sodium

EXCHANGES: **1 fruit**

Bread-and-Butter Pickle Relish

———◆———

The first year I grew zucchini, I planted six hills for just two people. Needless to say, I soon discovered how prolific squash plants could be, and I began looking for creative ways of using zucchini. After my mother mentioned using them in cucumber pickle recipes, I decided to try making relish. I loved it! The zucchini could be cut up much faster than cucumbers, and I soon made enough to last two years. I usually cut up the zucchini the night before and leave it to soak, and then I cook and pack the jars the next morning.

Try this relish in potato and pasta salad recipes. It is wonderful.

5 lb. unpeeled tender zucchini, ends removed, and cut
  into ¼-inch cubes
½ c. pickling salt
6 c. cider vinegar
4 c. sugar
2 tsp. celery seed
1 Tbsp. mustard seed
½ Tbsp. turmeric

Place zucchini in large bowl, and cover with cold water. Stir in salt, and let sit for at least 2 hours. Drain thoroughly.

Add vinegar, sugar, celery seed, mustard seed, and turmeric to large pot, and bring to a boil. Add zucchini, and let liquid return to boil. Reduce heat to simmer, and continue to cook 3–4 more minutes.

Pack zucchini in sterile jars to within ¼ inch of top, and then add syrup to cover. Seal, and process in boiling water bath 15–20 minutes. Remove from water, and check seals. (Read basic cookbook for instructions if canning is unfamiliar to you.)

YIELD: 6 pt.

Each 1 Tbsp. serving: Approx. 21 calories, 0.1 g fat (4.3% calories from fat), 0 g saturated fat, 0 g polyunsaturated fat, 0 g monounsaturated fat, 0 mg cholesterol, 5.1 g carbohydrate, 0.1 g protein, 57 mg sodium

EXCHANGES: ⅓ fruit

Herb and Garlic Vinegar

◆

Here's a fun vinegar to use when making vinaigrette to use as a salad dressing. It's also fun to give for gifts, especially when given in a pretty bottle with cork.

    2 c. cider vinegar or red wine vinegar
    2 sprigs fresh basil
    2 sprigs fresh oregano
    6 cloves garlic, mashed and peeled
    6 whole black peppercorns

In small saucepan, heat vinegar just to simmer. (Do not boil.) Place rest of ingredients in cruet or bottle, and pour hot vinegar into bottle. Cork or cover tightly. Let sit at room temperature 24 hours. At this point, you may want to remove herbs and garlic, or you may leave them in if vinegar will be used soon.

YIELD: 2 c.

Each 1 Tbsp. serving: 3 calories, 0 g fat (0% calories from fat), 0 g saturated fat, 0 g polyunsaturated fat, 0 g monounsaturated fat, 0 mg cholesterol, 0.9 g carbohydrate, 0 g protein, 0 mg sodium

EXCHANGES: Free

Hot Pepper Vinegar

◆

Here's a vinegar that will add zip to your salads and cooked greens. I like to leave one pepper in the bottle for decoration.

2 c. cider vinegar
4–6 dried hot red peppers

Heat vinegar to a simmer, but do not boil. Place peppers in cruet or corked bottle, and pour hot vinegar into bottle. Cork or close tightly, and let sit at room temperature 6 hours. Taste vinegar and remove peppers if vinegar is spicy enough. If not, leave them in.

YIELD: 2c.

Each 1 Tbsp. serving: 3 calories, 0 g fat (0% calories from fat), 0 g saturated fat, 0 g polyunsaturated fat, 0 g monounsaturated fat, 0 mg cholesterol, 0.9 g carbohydrate, 0 g protein, 0 mg sodium

EXCHANGES: Free

SALAD DRESSINGS

Herbed Vinaigrette

———◆———

Use your own Herb and Garlic Vinegar (page 283) in this dressing, if you wish. By experimenting with different herbs and vinegars, you will soon come up with a vinaigrette that's all your own.

1 c. cider vinegar or Herb and Garlic Vinegar
½ c. water
1 tsp. dried oregano or 1 Tbsp. finely chopped fresh
   oregano
1 tsp. dried basil or 1 Tbsp. finely chopped fresh basil
⅛ tsp. ground black pepper
⅛ tsp. salt
Optional: 1 tsp. to 1 Tbsp. sugar
Optional: 1 clove garlic, pressed
2 Tbsp. good-quality olive oil

Place vinegar, water, herbs, and seasonings in cruet. Add olive oil, and shake well. Refrigerate until flavors blend. Always shake well before using.

YIELD: Approx. 1½ c.

Each 1 Tbsp. serving: 15 calories, 1.4 g fat, 0.2 g saturated fat, 0.1 g polyunsaturated fat, 1.0 g monounsaturated fat, 0 mg cholesterol, 0.9 g carbohydrate, 0 g protein, 14 mg sodium

EXCHANGES: Free

Tomato-Basil Vinaigrette

◆

Here is a nice light vinaigrette, especially delicious when made with vine-ripened tomatoes.

    1 medium tomato, quartered
    ¼ tsp. salt
    1 Tbsp. cider vinegar
    4 peppercorns or pinch ground black pepper
    2 tsp. sugar
    1 small clove garlic
    6 fresh basil leaves or 2 tsp. dried basil

Place tomato, salt, vinegar, peppercorns, sugar, and garlic in bowl of food processor or blender and process until tomato is well blended. Add basil leaves, and process until basil leaves are well chopped. Store in refrigerator.

YIELD: Approx. ¾ c.

Each 1 Tbsp. serving: 5 calories, <0.1 g fat (4% calories from fat), 0 g saturated fat, 0 g polyunsaturated fat, 0 g monounsaturated fat, 0 mg cholesterol, 1.2 g carbohydrate, 0.1 g protein, 45 mg sodium

EXCHANGES: Free

Garlic-Peppercorn Dressing

———— ◆ ————

This dressing is similar to ranch dressing. Use yogurt or fat-free sour cream, depending on which flavor you prefer.

½ c. plus 1½ c. plain nonfat yogurt or fat-free sour cream
1 clove garlic
1 small onion, quartered
½ tsp. salt
12 black peppercorns or ¼ tsp. ground black pepper

Scoop the ½ c. yogurt into bowl of blender or food processor. Add garlic, onion, salt, and peppercorns. Blend or process 1–2 minutes, until smooth, and then stir the remaining 1½ c. yogurt in by hand. Refrigerate until ready to use.

YIELD: Approx. 2 c.

Each 1 Tbsp. serving: 9 calories, <0.1 g total fat (3% calories from fat), 0 g saturated fat, 0 g polyunsaturated fat, 0 g monounsaturated fat, 0 mg cholesterol, 1.3 g carbohydrate, 0.9 g protein, 44 mg sodium

EXCHANGES: Free

Index